ORL

OXFORD RHEUMATOLOGY LIBRARY

Gout

O R L

OXFORD RHEUMATOLOGY LIBRARY

Gout

Nicola Dalbeth

Department of Medicine, University of Auckland, Auckland, New Zealand

Lisa Stamp

Department of Medicine, University of Otago, Christchurch, New Zealand

Tony Merriman

Biochemistry Department, School of Medical Sciences,
University of Otago, Dunedin, New Zealand

OXFORD
UNIVERSITY PRESS

OXFORD
UNIVERSITY PRESS

Great Clarendon Street, Oxford, OX2 6DP,
United Kingdom

Oxford University Press is a department of the University of Oxford.
It furthers the University's objective of excellence in research, scholarship,
and education by publishing worldwide. Oxford is a registered trade mark of
Oxford University Press in the UK and in certain other countries

First Edition published in 2016

Impression: 1

Published in the United States of America by Oxford University Press
198 Madison Avenue, New York, NY 10016, United States of America

British Library Cataloguing in Publication Data

Data available

Library of Congress Control Number: 2015949836

ISBN 978–0–19–874831–1

Printed and bound in Great Britian by
Clays Ltd, St Ives plc

Contents

Symbols and Abbreviations

&	and
=	equal to
<	less than
>	greater than
≤	equal to or less than
≥	equal to or greater than
ACE	angiotensin-converting enzyme
ACR	American College of Rheumatology
AGREE	Acute Gout Flare Receiving Colchicine Evaluation
AHS	allopurinol hypersensitivity syndrome
APRT	adenine phosphoribosyltransferase
ASC	apoptosis-associated speck-like protein
ATP	adenosine triphosphate
BMI	body mass index
BSR	British Society for Rheumatology
CI	confidence interval
CK	creatine kinase
CKD	chronic kidney disease
COX	cyclo-oxygenase
CPP	calcium pyrophosphate
CPPD	calcium pyrophosphate deposition
CrCL	creatinine clearance
CT	computed tomography
CVD	cardiovascular disease
d	day
DECT	dual energy CT
dL	decilitre
DRESS	drug reaction with eosinophilia and systemic symptoms
eGFR	estimated GFR
ESCISIT	EULAR Standing Committee for International Clinical Studies Including Therapeutic
eSNP	expression SNP
EULAR	European League Against Rheumatism

FBC	full blood count
FDA	Food and Drug Administration
FEUA	fractional excretion of uric acid
g	gram
G6PD	glucose-6-phosphate dehydrogenase
GAQ2.0	Gout Assessment Questionnaire version 2
GCKR	glucokinase regulatory
GFR	glomerular filtration rate
GI	gastrointestinal
GMP	guanosine monophosphate
GOMRICS	GOut MRI Cartilage Score
Gp	glycoprotein
GTP	guanosine triphosphate
GWAS	genome-wide association study
H^2	broad-sense heritability
HFI	hereditary fructose intolerance
HLF	hepatic leukemia factor
HPRT	hypoxanthine-guanine phosphoribosyltransferase
HR	hazard ratio
IA	intra-articular
IgA	immunoglobin A
IgG	immunoglobin G
IL	interleukin
IM	intra-muscular
IMP	inosine monophosphate
INR	international normalized ratio
IV	intravenous
kb	kilo-base
kg	kilogram
L	litre
LRP2	lipoprotein receptor–related protein 2
m	metre
mg	milligram
MI	myocardial infarction
µm	micron
mm	millimetre
mmHg	millimetre of mercury
mmol	millimole
MRI	magnetic resonance imaging
MSU	monosodium urate

MTPJ	metatarsophalangeal joint
MyD88	myeloid-dependent factor 88
NET	neutrophil extracellular traps
NHANES	National Health and Nutrition Examination Survey
NSAID	non-steroidal anti-inflammatory drug
OMERACT	Outcomes in Rheumatology Clinical Trials
OR	odds ratio
p	probability
PNP	purine nucleotide phosphorylase
PRPP	phosphoribosyl pyrophosphate
RA	rheumatoid arthritis
RAMRIS	Rheumatoid Arthritis Magnetic Resonance Imaging System
RR	relative risk
SCAR	severe cutaneous adverse reaction
SD	standard deviation
SJS/TEN	Stevens Johnson/toxic epidermal necrolysis
SNP	single nucleotide polymorphism
SSB	sugar-sweetened beverages
SU	serum urate
SUGAR	Study for Updated Gout Classification Criteria
TLR	toll-like receptor
UGT	uridine diphosphate-glucuronosyltransferase
UK	United Kingdom
ULT	urate-lowering therapy
US	ultrasonography
UUE	urinary uric acid excretion
VLDL	very low density lipoprotein

Chapter 1

Introduction to gout

Key points

- Gout is a common and treatable cause of musculoskeletal disability.
- There have been major advances in scientific understanding and treatment of gout in the last decade.
- Despite these advances, gout is often neglected and poorly managed.
- This handbook summarizes recent progress and provides a framework for effective gout management.

Gout is the most common form of inflammatory arthritis in adults. The prevalence of gout is rising, and now affects approximately one in 25 adults in the United States. The impact of gout on the individual, family, and wider community occurs due to the disease itself and the frequent associated co-morbid conditions. This disease causes flares of severe joint pain, structural bone and cartilage damage, loss of participation, and disability. Gout is also strongly associated with other important chronic conditions such as hypertension, chronic kidney disease, coronary artery disease, and type 2 diabetes.

The last decade has seen major progress in our understanding of gout. Advances in the basic biology of disease have included the genetics of hyperuricaemia and gout, the physiology of renal urate transport, and the understanding of gut urate transport as a mediator of serum urate. New advanced imaging methods represent exciting non-invasive tools for gout diagnosis. These imaging methods have allowed novel insights into the natural history of disease and emphasized that gout is a chronic disease of monosodium urate (MSU) crystal deposition. New imaging tools are also included in the 2015 American College of Rheumatology (ACR)/European League Against Rheumatism (EULAR) gout classification criteria. The understanding of MSU crystal–induced NLRP3 inflammasome activation led to recognition that IL-1β is the central cytokine in acute gouty inflammation, which has translated into new therapies for treatment of acute gout flares. New urate-lowering drugs have been approved for the first time in half a century, providing wider treatment options than ever before. A number of other urate-lowering drugs are in pipeline development. The major rheumatology societies (ACR, EULAR, and the British Society for Rheumatology) have issued gout management guidelines. Although there are some regional differences, the central focus of all of these guidelines is long-term serum urate lowering.

Despite these exciting developments, gout remains a neglected condition in primary care, in rheumatology practice, and in basic and clinical research. Most people with gout do not receive effective treatment consistent with best-practice recommendations. Healthcare professionals, reflecting general public attitudes, often view gout as a humorous disease caused by personal excess. Such attitudes are an important barrier to empathic and effective management. Many other myths about gout management also exist, which create inconsistency, inadequate care, and confusion for people with gout.

Against this background of progress and challenges, we hope that readers will find this handbook to be a useful and up-to-date clinical resource on gout. We have focused on key aspects of the biology of the disease, relevant diagnostic tools, principles of gout management, and practical information to guide safe and effective prescribing of gout medications. We hope that this handbook will lead to updated knowledge, newfound enthusiasm for this disease, and, ultimately, improved management for many people with gout.

Chapter 2

Aetiopathogenesis

Key points

- The aetiopathogenesis of gout is initiated by urate overproduction and uric acid under-excretion leading to hyperuricaemia.
- Foods such as seafood, red meat, beer, and sugar-sweetened beverages contribute to overproduction.
- Under-excretion is caused by renal and gut uric acid transporters such as SLC2A9, ABCG2, and URAT1.
- In gout there is formation of monosodium urate (MSU) crystals in joints, with acute gouty arthritis mediated by the innate immune system in response to these crystals.
- Factors such as urate concentration, proteins present in synovial fluid, temperature, and pH control crystal nucleation and growth.
- Activation of the NLRP3 inflammasome by MSU crystals and production of interleukin-1β is central to acute gouty arthritis.
- Advanced gout occurs when there is chronic gouty arthritis and tophus formation, with the tophus being an organized immune tissue response to MSU crystals that involves both innate and adaptive immune cells.
- Progression through the gout checkpoints (hyperuricaemia, MSU crystal formation, and immune response) is governed by inherited genetic variants, lifetime environmental exposures, and their interaction.

The aetiopathogenesis of gout is dictated by several key checkpoints (see Figure 2.1): hyperuricaemia, formation of MSU crystals, and subsequent innate immune response (Merriman and Dalbeth 2011). Progression through these checkpoints is governed by inherited genetic variants, lifetime environmental exposures, and their interaction. Once hyperuricaemia exists, progression to gout can be regarded as four progressive phases: asymptomatic hyperuricaemia without evidence of MSU crystal deposition, hyperuricaemia with evidence of MSU crystal deposition, MSU crystal deposition with prior or current symptoms of acute gouty arthritis, and advanced gout with tophi (Dalbeth and Stamp 2014).

2.1 Urate

Urate, the ionized form of uric acid, is synthesized predominantly in the liver. In the absence of significant binding to plasma proteins (<4% under physiologic conditions), the majority of circulating urate is available for filtration as the un-ionized form (uric acid) present in normal acidic urine (pH ~5) at the renal glomerulus and available for unidirectional excretion through the gut. The solubility of urate, which constitutes 98% of urate/uric acid at the pH and sodium

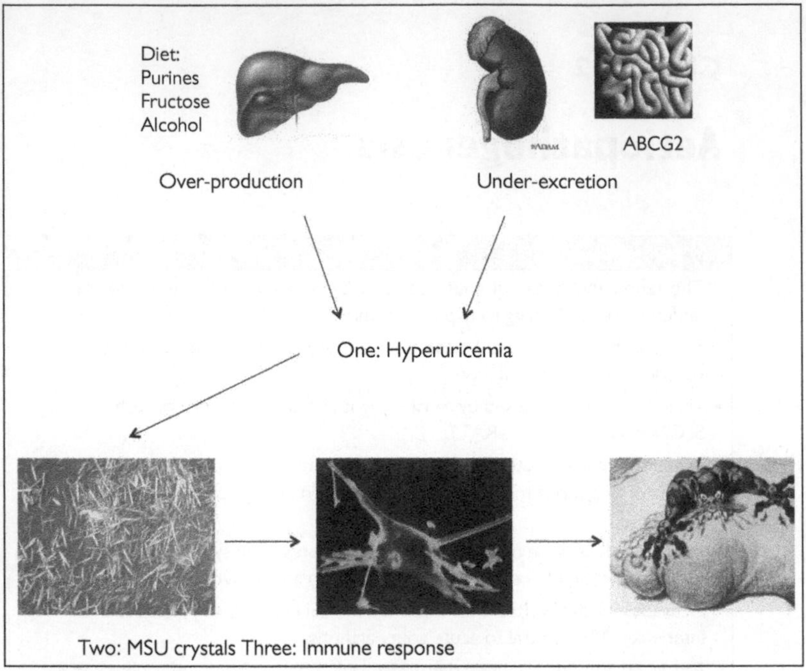

Figure 2.1 Key checkpoints in gout. One: a combination of overproduction and renal and gut under-excretion results in hyperuricaemia. Two: MSU crystals form in a minority of people with hyperuricaemia. Three: factors governing the innate immune response to MSU crystals.

concentration of serum, is relatively limited, around 0.40–0.41 mmol/L (~6.7 mg/dL). In supersaturation, urate precipitates in the form of MSU crystals.

Historically, research into urate has focused on its role as a cause of gout, and numerous observational studies have associated urate with co-morbid conditions (see Chapter 3). However, as discussed in Chapter 3, a possible causal role for urate in other pathology remains to be resolved. Before focusing on the role of urate in the pathogenesis of gout, it is therefore important to gain some perspective on reasons why humans have elevated levels of this metabolite.

Humans and the greater apes are unique in the animal kingdom in having elevated levels of urate (Chang 2014; Kratzer et al. 2014). The primary reason for this is a number of separate promoter and amino-acid sequence mutational events leading to the inactivation of the urate-degrading enzyme uricase during the evolution of hominoid primates. Uricase produces the more soluble compound and readily excreted compound allantoin. The presumption that the inactivation of uricase was the result of natural selection strongly supports the argument that individuals with a higher serum urate had an evolutionary advantage by a combination of metabolic advantage (enhanced conversion of fruit-derived fructose into fat), enhancing early hominid foraging and food intake, increasing blood pressure and blood flow to the enlarged brain in early bipedal hominids in a low-salt environment, a potent antioxidant and neuroprotectant, and an innate immune system stimulant in the crystalline form that is able to enhance response to infectious disease (Shi et al. 2010). The complex suite of renal uric acid–handling molecules that mediate the reuptake of 90% of filtered uric acid that humans have acquired—the 'transportasome'—is also consistent with a beneficial role for urate in human physiology.

2.1.1 **Urate production**

Urate overproduction is one established cause of hyperuricaemia. Urate is a catabolic product of purine metabolism (Figure 2.2), with production a result of dietary purine intake, hepatic metabolism of sugars and alcohol, disorders associated with high cellular turnover, and rare genetic disorders disrupting the endogenous metabolism of purines. It is important to note that the concept of urate overproduction has been redefined as genuine overproduction (outlined later) and overproduction caused by reduced gut excretion of uric acid by genetically inherited variants in the ABCG2 transporter (see also Chapter 4) (Ichida et al. 2012).

Epidemiological studies have associated foods with high purine content (such as red meat) with elevated urate levels and risk of gout; administration of certain purines elevates serum urate levels, with increased elevation in people with gout (Clifford et al. 1976). Similarly, sugar consumption, particularly in the form of sugar-sweetened beverages, and alcohol consumption are associated with increased urate and risk of gout. Oral administration of alcohol and fructose increases serum urate at least partly by depletion of ATP and generation of AMP during hepatic processing (Johnson et al. 2009), which is processed by adenosine deaminase into IMP and ultimately into urate (Figure 2.2). Beer is more strongly associated with increased urate and risk of gout than other alcoholic beverages, with the increased purine (guanosine) content of beer speculated to augment the direct effect of ethanol. Elevated urate levels from catabolism of nucleic acids (purines) is a feature of tumour lysis syndrome.

Finally, there are rare genetic causes of urate overproduction (Merriman and Dalbeth 2011) (see also Chapter 4). Examples are mutations in hypoxanthine-guanine phosphoribosyltransferase (involved in the purine salvage pathway) deficiency and phosphoribosylpyrophosphate synthetase (involved in the purine de novo synthesis pathway) superactivity, both of which can cause urate overproduction.

2.1.2 **Urate under-excretion**

Approximately two-thirds of uric acid excretion occurs through the kidney, with the remainder through the gastrointestinal tract.

2.1.2.1 *Renal excretion of uric acid*

Renal excretion of uric acid is measured by fractional excretion of uric acid (FEUA), which is the ratio of uric acid excreted to creatinine excreted. Reference intervals in Europeans are 7–9.5% for men, 10–14% for women, and 15–22% for children. Reduced FEUA is well established as a cause of hyperuricaemia. For example, normouricaemic and gouty Māori men (drawn from the hyperuricaemic Māori [Polynesian] population of New Zealand) have reduced FEUA compared to European men (4.9 vs 8.1% and 3.6 vs 5.6%, respectively; Gibson et al. 1984), and normouricaemic women have increased FEUA compared to men (9.7 vs 4.9% in Polynesians and 12.8 vs 8.1% in Europeans).

The textbook model of renal uric acid excretion consists of four steps: glomerular filtration, reabsorption from this filtrate, subsequent secretion, and post-secretory reabsorption (Roch-Ramel and Guisan 1999), leading to the excretion of ~10% of the uric acid initially filtered. The four-step model has been critically reviewed (Mandal and Mount 2015). Physiological studies in species that reabsorb more uric acid support the coexistence of secretion and reabsorption along the entire proximal tubule (Mandal and Mount 2015). Further, it has been observed that the four-component model was based on a conclusion that pyrazinamide inhibited secretion of uric acid, whereas it appears to enhance reabsorption via URAT1.

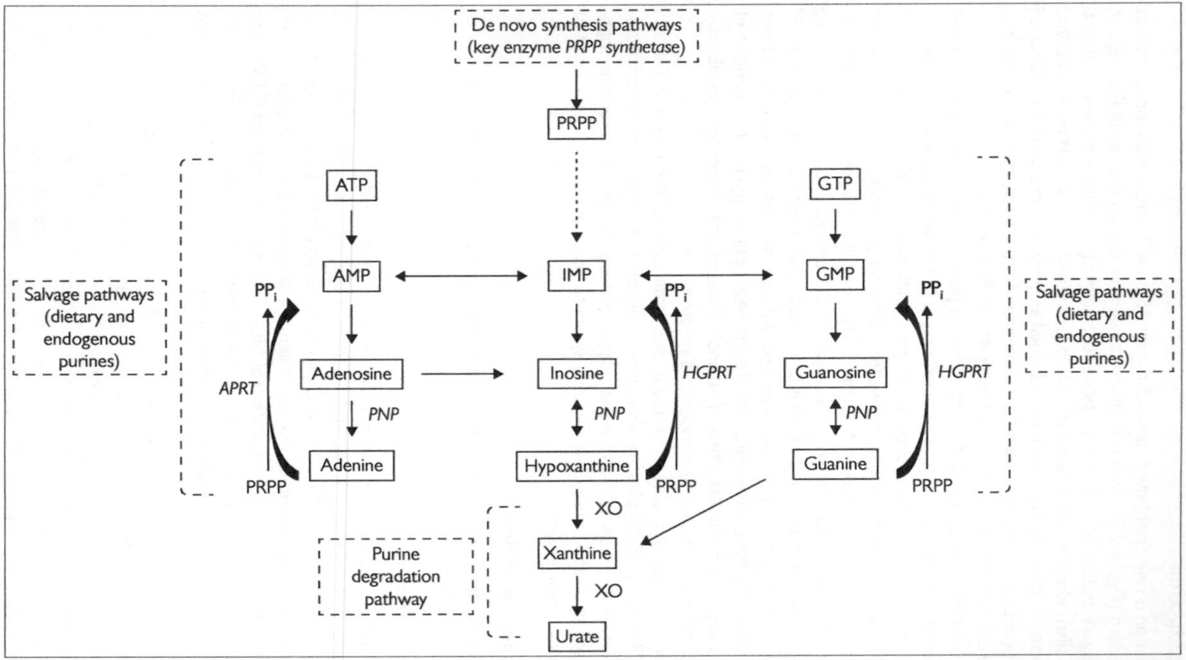

Figure 2.2 Urate production pathways. The de novo synthesis starts with 5′-phosphoribosyl 1-pyrophosphate (PRPP), which is produced by addition of a further phosphate group from adenosine triphosphate (ATP) to the modified sugar ribose-5-phosphate (ribose-5-P). This step is performed by the family of PRPP synthetase enzymes. In addition, purine bases derived from tissue nucleic acids are reutilized through the salvage pathway. The enzyme hypoxanthine-guanine phosphoribosyltransferase (HPRT) salvages hypoxanthine to inosine monophosphate (IMP) and guanine to guanosine monophosphate (GMP). Other abbreviations: APRT, adenine phosphoribosyltransferase; GTP, guanosine triphosphate; PNP, purine nucleotide phosphorylase.

Reproduced from Dalbeth, N., Pathological basis of hyperuricemia and gout, Gout, 2013, with permission from Future Medicine LTD.

The renal handling of uric acid is controlled by a complex array of transporters and regulatory/accessory molecules collectively termed the 'uric acid transportasome' (Anzai et al. 2012; Dalbeth and Merriman 2009; Mandal and Mount 2015) (see Figure 2.3). Comprehensively reviewed elsewhere (Mandal and Mount 2015), the key transporters can be grouped into reabsorptive uric acid-anion exchangers (URAT1/SLC22A12, OAT4/SLC22A11, OAT10/SLC22A3), the reabsorptive GLUT9/SLC2A9 uric acid transporter, secretory anion exchangers transporters (OAT1, OAT2, OAT3), sodium-phosphate transporter proteins (NPT1/SLC17A1, NPT4/SLC17A3), and the ATP-driven secretory efflux pump, MRP4/ABCC4. The intracellular concentration of anions is important for uric acid transport, which is largely dependent on sodium-dependent absorption from the glomerular filtrate. Two sodium-dependent monocarboxylate anion cotransporters (SMCT1/SLC5A8, SMCT2/SLC5A12) interact with URAT1. Important regulatory proteins are PDZK1 and NHERF1, which contain a 'PDZ' domain interaction motif. These proteins regulate the trafficking and activity of proteins, including SLC22 and ABC uric acid transporters, involved in renal proximal tubule transport. Genome-wide and candidate gene association studies have emphasized the importance of *SLC2A9* and *ABCG2* in determining variability between individuals in susceptibility to hyperuricaemia (Köttgen et al. 2013; Phipps-Green et al. 2014). Weaker genetic associations are evident with *SLC22A11*, *SLC22A12*, *SLC17A1*, *SLC17A3*, and *PDZK1*.

The abolition of renal reabsorption of uric acid in hypouricaemic patients with homozygous inactivating mutations in *SLC2A9* (Dinour et al. 2010), and the extremely strong association of common variants in *SLC2A9* with hyperuricaemia and common gout (Köttgen et al. 2013) emphasize the important role of GLUT9 in control of urate levels. (The causal variants in *SLC2A9* have yet to be identified, but presumably are gain-of-function via causing increased expression of an isoform of GLUT9 on the apical membrane of the proximal tubule; Doring et al. 2008; Merriman and Dalbeth 2011). Isoforms are generated from the same gene with one missing 31 N-terminal residues that is expressed on the apical membrane, and the full-length protein is expressed on the basolateral membrane. GLUT9 has a transmembrance motif conserved with other GLUT transporters, which should confer the ability to transport fructose in exchange for uric acid, although this remains to be universally demonstrated (Mandal and Mount 2015). The activity of GLUT9 is inhibited to a limited extent by the uricosuric drug benzbromarone and not at all by probenecid. URAT1 is the dominant apical uric acid exchanger in the proximal tubule, exchanging secreted uric acid for anions such as lactate, butyrate, and nicotinate, with the uricosuric drugs benzbromarone and probenecid strong inhibitors.

2.1.2.2 *Clinical aspects of renal uric acid excretion*

The renal transport physiology has clinical consequences (Mandal and Mount 2015). Hyperuricaemia occurs with increased concentration of β-hydroxybutyrate and acetoacetate in diabetic ketoacidosis, with starvation ketosis and increased lactate (a consequence of alcohol consumption) increasing reabsorption of uric acid—probably contributing to the association between hyperuricaemia and alcohol. The use of drugs such as nicotinic acid and pyrazinamide can be complicated by hyperuricaemia.

Urate levels and the risk of incident gout are increased by the use of diuretics, particularly thiazide and loop diuretics. The molecular explanation for this association is not understood, with circulating volume depletion and reduced renal blood flow proposed to influence peritubular factors and increase reabsorption. An unreplicated epidemiological nonadditive interaction between genetic variation in the GLUT9 and OAT4 transporters and diuretics in influencing risk of incident gout in hypertensive individuals (see Chapter 4) suggests that physiological studies of the influence of diuretics on the function of uric acid transporters may provide mechanistic insight and perhaps allow development of uricosuric diuretics. Losartan is hypouricaemic and protective of incident gout, with inhibition of the reabsorptive activity of

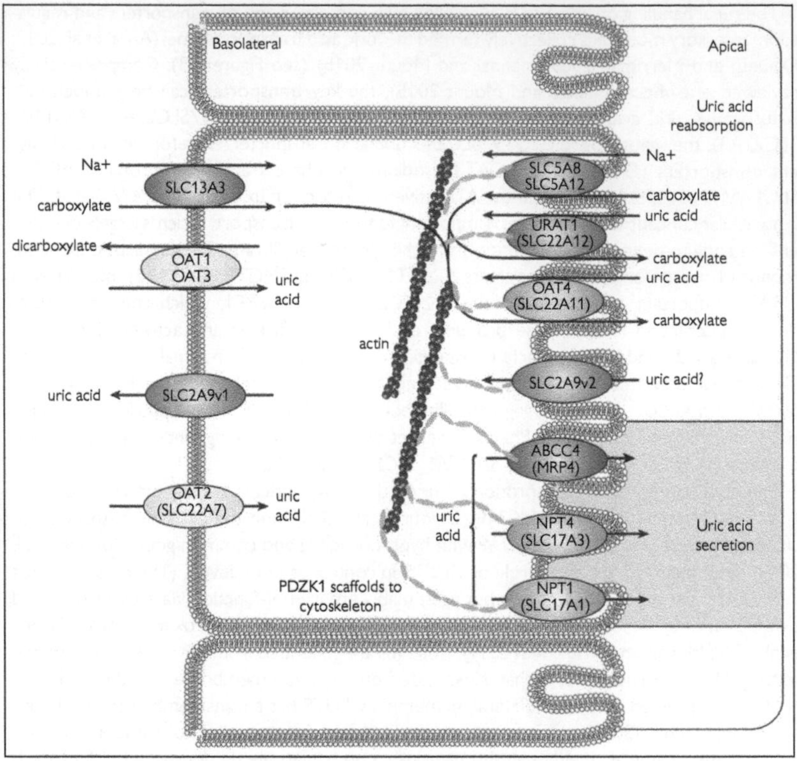

Figure 2.3 The uric acid transportasome. Current understanding of uric acid transport in the proximal renal tubule. Carboxylates accumulate in the tubular cell through sodium-dependent monocarboxylate transporters SLC5A8 and SLC5A12, and through SLC13A3. Uric acid enters the cell in exchange for carboxylate via apical URAT1 and apical OAT4. Apical SLC2A9v2 plays a significant role in uric acid reabsorption, the reabsorbed uric acid exiting the cell through basolateral SLC2A9v1. For efflux of uric acid into the lumen, MRP4 and voltage-driven organic anion transporters (NPT1/NPT4) are candidates. OAT1 and OAT3 are known to transport uric acid, although the direction of transport is not clear. PDZK1 is a scaffolding protein involved in assembly of a transporter complex in the apical membrane. Genetic variation in SLC2A9, URAT1, NPT1/NPT4, OAT4, and PDZK1 is associated with serum urate levels and gout.

URAT1 a likely mechanism. Finally, epidemiological and clinical data demonstrating interaction between sugar exposure and genetic variation in GLUT9 (which also transports hexose sugars) suggest a direct influence of fructose and glucose on uric acid transport.

2.1.2.3 *Gut excretion of uric acid*

A number of functional variations in ABCG2 reduce the activity of this secretory transporter and are associated with hyperuricaemia and gout. Unexpectedly, two urate-increasing genetic variants in *ABCG2* (Q141K and Q126X) increase urinary uric acid excretion in humans, and in mice, an *Abcg2*-knockout also showed increased renal but decreased gut uric acid excretion (Ichida et al. 2012). The urate-increasing allele at *Q141K* (141K) has been associated with a reduced increase in serum urate and glucose in response to a fructose load. Collectively, these results show that the urate-increasing variant at ABCG2 does not act via direct effects on renal uric acid transport, but rather through increased gut excretion. Ichida et al. (2012) proposed that ABCG2 defines one of the three pathways contributing to hyperuricaemia; namely, extra-renal uric acid under-excretion. With the caveat that results from *Slc2Aa9*-inactivation studies in the mouse can be extrapolated to humans only with much caution (given the presence of active urate oxidase [uricase] in mice), a recent study demonstrates that SLC2A9 could be an important basolateral uric acid efflux transporter into the gut enterocyte in humans (DeBosch et al. 2014).

2.2 Formation of MSU crystals

Acute gouty arthritis is a response to the nucleation and growth of MSU crystals in hyperuricaemia. Given that only 24% of asymptomatic individuals with serum urate >0.54 mmol/L have evidence of MSU crystal deposition, and that deposition occurs preferentially at specific sites—for example, the first metatarsophalangeal joint, Achilles and patellar tendons—it is clear that urate-independent factors contribute to MSU crystallization (Chhana et al. 2015). The factors would be expected to be those influencing urate solubility (causing supersaturation), nucleation, and crystal growth.

Reviewed in Chhana et al. (2015), the solubility of urate is influenced by temperature (decreased temperature reduces solubility), pH (close to neutrality, pH 7–8, reduces solubility), and sodium chloride (increased concentration reduces solubility). The solubility of urate at physiological temperature and sodium levels has been estimated at 0.404 mmol/L. Cartilage matrix components also influence solubility, with structurally intact protein polysaccharides and proteoglycans increasing solubility. Factors derived from plasma and synovial fluid can also influence the solubility of urate, although the nature of these factors is currently unclear (Chhana et al. 2015).

Nucleation, the appearance of new MSU crystals, is hypothesized to occur when MSU molecules have clustered and reached a critical stable mass and are no longer susceptible to dissolution within the solvent. In-vitro studies indicate that elevated urate and Na^+ concentrations are important (reviewed in Chhana et al. 2015). However, in vivo MSU nucleation is likely to be induced by connective tissue factors and proteins, given that they generally form and deposit on cartilage. Gouty synovial fluid speeds up the appearance of, and increases the total amount of, MSU crystals formed. High molecular weight proteins, such as serum albumin, globulins, and type I collagen, increase MSU nucleation in vitro, and there is evidence that IgG antibodies, which are present in gouty synovial fluid, can enhance nucleation. Further, IgG antibodies can be induced from injection of rabbits with MSU crystals, but not with other types of crystals.

Once MSU crystals are present, there are factors that influence the rate of growth. One such factor is increased urate concentration. Interestingly, MSU crystals grown in vitro have a smaller average and tighter range of length when exposed to human serum or synovial fluid when compared to crystals grown in the absence of any additional factors. A case report of a male gout patient with mitochondriopathy in Kearns-Sayre syndrome was described in which MSU crystals alone failed to induce the inflammatory response, although the circulating serum urate concentration was 0.92 mmol/L (Jansen et al. 2014). This person had large MSU crystals that were less immunogenic and exhibited little synergy with toll-like receptor 2 (TLR2) agonists, a response that was hypothesized to be due to different crystal conformational or chemicophysical properties on exposure to C16.0 or pam-3-cys compounds. This report supports the finding that along with raised serum urate levels, specific stereochemical/conformational crystal properties are needed for acute gouty arthritis.

2.3 The immune response to MSU crystals

The acute gouty flare is a sterile inflammatory response to MSU crystals that, in the absence of intervention, resolves within a 7–10 day period. Key inflammatory cells are neutrophils, with macrophages, mast cells, and endothelial cells also important (Liu-Bryan and Terkeltaub 2011). At the molecular level, production of interleukin-1β (IL-1β) via MSU crystal activation of the caspase recruitment domain-containing protein 8 (CARD8) NOD-like receptor pyrin-containing 3 (NLRP3) inflammasome is central to acute gouty arthritis (see Figure 2.4). Evidence is accumulating that fatty acid metabolites can modulate this response.

Initiation of the acute gouty flare occurs when MSU crystals are phagocytosed by resident macrophages, resulting in NLRP3 inflammasome activation. Expression of the toll-like receptors 2 and 4 in a functional complex involving CD14 and leukocyte β integrins are important in inflammasome activation, with a dependence on myeloid-dependent factor 88 (MyD88) expression and signalling. The NLRP3 protein forms the inflammasome with its adaptor protein ASC (apoptosis-associated speck-like protein). Induction of the NLRP3 inflammasome involves inactivation of the α-tubulin deacetylase sirtuin 2 via disruption of mitochodrial homeostasis.

The acetylated α-tubulin then mediates the transport of mitochondrial-bound ASC to NLRP3 on the endoplasmic reticulum, a process that is inhibited by colchicine (Misawa et al. 2013). Inflammasome activation, which requires reactive oxygen species, results in cleavage of pro-IL-1β into mature IL-1β by caspase-1, that is recruited and activated by the inflammasome. The MyD88-dependent signalling results in NF-κB activation, which also leads to expression of other pro-inflammatory cytokines, such as TNF-α, IL-6, and IL-8 (Liu-Bryan et al. 2005).

Alongside MSU crystals, a second signal is required for the production of mature IL-1β. One such signal comes from long-chain free fatty acids (Joosten et al. 2010). This second signal could be related to the well-established, but poorly understood in a mechanistic sense, dietary triggers of acute gout attacks, including seafood, alcohol, and red meat. It is interesting that the short-chain butyric acid inhibits pro-IL-1β production at the transcriptional level, probably via influencing histone deacetylation.

Once initiated by the reaction of monocytes to MSU crystals, the acute gouty attack is amplified by vascular endothelial cell activation in response to pro-inflammatory cytokines (e.g. IL-1β), which allows increased permeability of tissues to leukocytes. This is aided by expression of adhesion molecules (such as intracellular and vascular adhesion 1 molecules) and generation of chemokines, such as S100A8/A9 and IL-8. The gouty attack is further amplified by the involvement of neutrophils via interaction with MSU crystals, leading to the release of a host of other pro-inflammatory cytokines, chemokines, and other factors, such as reactive oxygen species, prostaglandin E2, and lysosomal enzymes.

In the resolution phase, TGFβ1 produced after apoptosis and noninflammatory phagocytosis of neutrophils suppresses further pro-inflammatory cytokine release by MSU-activated monocytes. The anti-inflammatory cytokines IL-1RA and IL-10 are also present at high concentrations in the synovial fluid during acute gout. More recently an important resolution mechanism has been revealed; namely, the antimicrobial 'neutrophil extracellular traps' (NETs) structures comprising DNA, histones, granular enzymes, and antimicrobial peptides. When this occurs, the cells undergo 'NETosis', which is a cell-death pathway distinct from apoptosis and necrosis, and dependent on the presence of reactive oxygen species (Fuchs et al. 2007). At the high neutrophil densities present during an acute gout attack, the NETs also bind and degrade pro-inflammatory mediators (Schauer et al. 2014).

During intercritical gout there must exist homeostasis between MSU crystals and the innate immune system, as crystals are present in individuals who have previously had gout attacks. The NETosis pathway may contribute to suppression of the monocyte response to MSU crystals. However, there is evidence that protein coating of MSU crystals can modulate the immune response. IgG has a pro-inflammatory effect and apolipoprotein B (apo B) has been linked with down-regulation of the innate immune system and the resolution phase of acute gout. When coating MSU crystals, apo B suppresses neutrophil activation, which is consistent with the clinical observation that apo B coats MSU crystals only when inflammation subsides in gout.

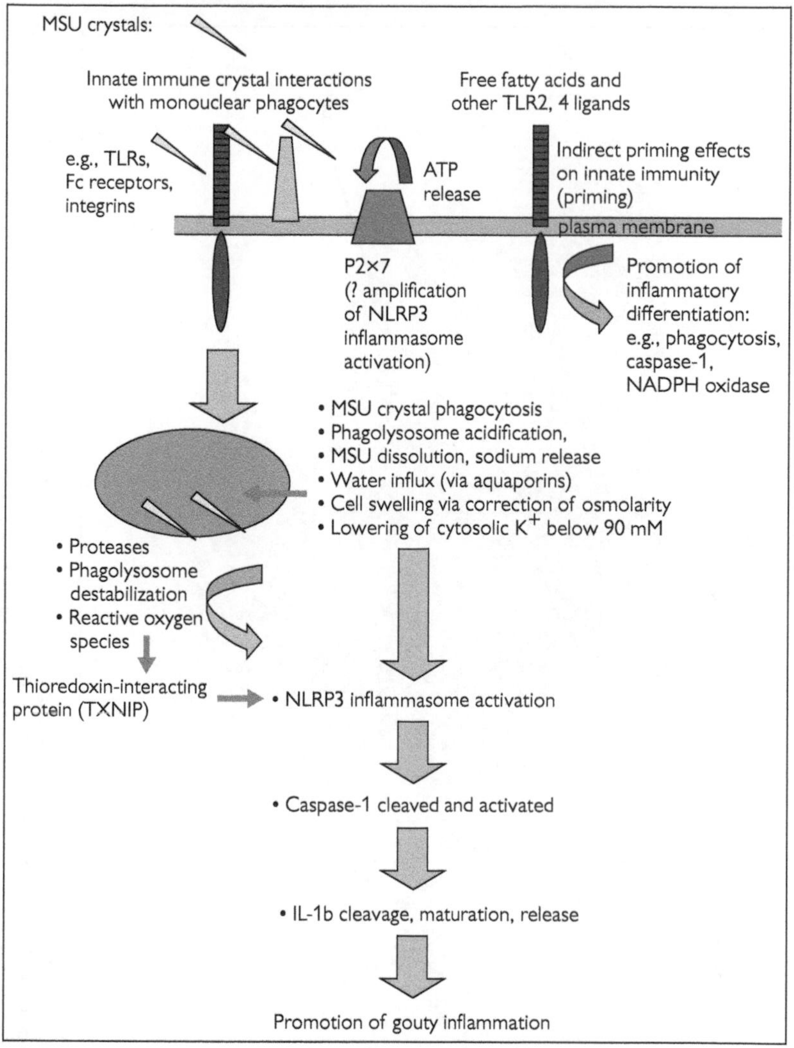

Figure 2.4 Innate immune activation of inflammation by MSU crystals: NLRP3 (cryopyrin) inflammasome, and interleukin (IL)-1β processing and secretion. MSU crystals perturb membranes and engage and cluster mobile membrane proteins at the macrophage surface, mediated by Fc receptors, integrins, as well the toll-like receptors TLR2 and TLR4 and associated MYD88 signalling. Priming of MSU crystal–induced macrophage activation by TLR2 ligand free fatty acids is also illustrated. Crystal uptake, and associated reactive oxygen species generation, protease release from phagolysosomes, sodium release from MSU crystal dissolution in phagolysosomes (and lowering of cytosolic calcium via consequent water influx, as well as P2X7-mediated K+ efflux), and recruitment of TXNIP, synergistically promote activation of the NLRP3 inflammasome. Consequent endoproteolytic activation of caspase-1 stimulates pro-IL-1β maturation, and results in secretion of mature IL-1β. *MyD88*: myeloid differentiation primary response gene 88; NLRP: Nacht domain, leucine-rich repeat- and PYD-containing protein; TLR: toll-like receptor.

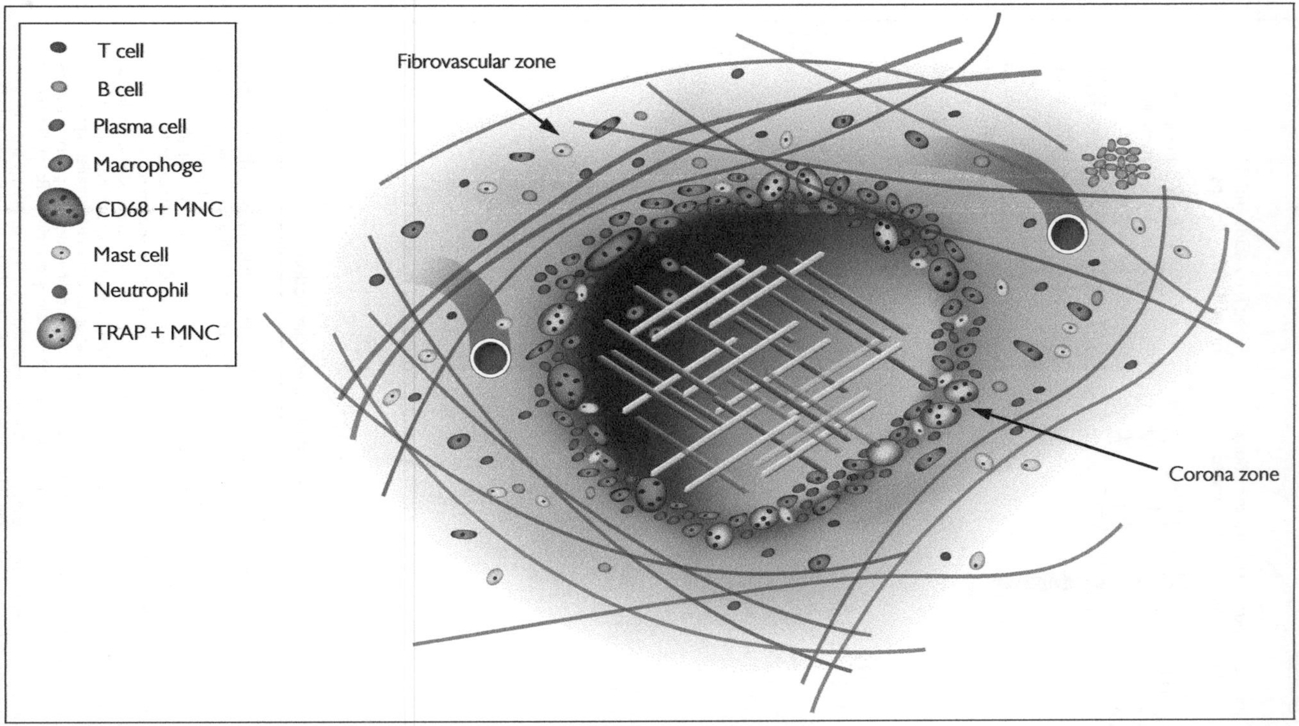

Figure 2.5 A cellular model of the gouty tophus. Cells are depicted in the corona and fibrovascular zones based on the type and number of cells identified by quantitative immunohistochemistry. MNC: mononuclear cells; TRAP: tartrate-resistant acid phosphatase.

Reprinted with permission from Cellular characterization of the gouty tophus: a quantitative analysis, Dalbeth, N, et al. Arthritis Rheum, 62, 1549–56. Copyright 2010 with permission from John Wiley and Sons Ltd.

Apolipoprotein E (apo E) also binds MSU crystals in vivo, and MSU crystal–bound apo E suppresses crystal–induced neutrophil activation in vitro. Apolipoproteins B and E are components of very low density lipoprotein (VLDL), and these MSU crystal–associated immune modulatory effects could be connected to the association of gout with type IV hyperlipoproteinemia (elevated VLDL) (Rasheed et al. 2013).

2.4 Chronic gout and tophus formation

Advanced gout occurs when there is persistent gouty arthritis and tophus. Aside from the direct contribution of hyperuricaemia to MSU crystal formation, the production of IL-1ß can be potentiated by soluble urate in a mechanism involving epigenetic reprogramming of monocytes (Crişan et al. 2015). This suggests a role for hyperuricaemia in potentiating chronic gouty inflammation. The tophus is an organized immune tissue response to MSU crystals that involves both innate and adaptive immune cells (see Figure 2.5) (Dalbeth et al. 2010). Both pro-inflammatory IL-1ß and anti-inflammatory TBF-ß1 are coexpressed in the tophus, implying an ongoing state of chronic MSU crystal–stimulated inflammation and attempted resolution (Dalbeth et al. 2010). Interleukin-1ß-producing macrophages are correlated with the formation of the tophus, suggesting that IL-1ß is required for formation (Dalbeth et al. 2010), consistent with the central role for this cytokine in formation of granulomas in other diseases (e.g. rheumatoid arthritis and tuberculosis). The presence of adaptive immune plasma and B cells may reflect their production of IgG which is implicated in MSU crystal formation and innate immune response (see the previous discussion) (Dalbeth et al. 2010). NETosis may play a role in tophus formation by organizing MSU crystals in a noninflammatory state and developing the crystal core with a subsequent dampening of the immune response. This would be consistent with the usual presentation of tophi as noninflammatory subcutaneous nodules.

References

Anzai N, et al. (2012). Recent advances in renal urate transport: characterization of candidate transporters indicated by genome-wide association studies. *Clinical and Experimental Nephrology*, 16, 89–95.

Chang BSW (2014). Ancient insights into uric acid metabolism in primates. *Proceedings of the National Academy of Sciences*, 111, 3657–58.

Chhana A, Lee G, Dalbeth N (2015). Factors influencing the crystallization of monosodium urate: a systematic literature review. BMC Musculoskelet Disord. 2015 Oct 14;16(1):296.

Clifford AJ, et al. (1976). Effect of oral purines on serum and urinary uric acid of normal, hyperuricemic and gouty humans. *Journal of Nutrition*, 106, 428–34.

Crişan TO, et al. (2015). Soluble uric acid primes TLR-induced proinflammatory cytokine production by human primary cells via inhibition of IL-1Ra. *Annals of the Rheumatic Diseases*. doi: 10.1136/annrheumdis-2014-206564

Dalbeth N (2013). The pathological basis of hyperuricaemia and gout. In N Dalbeth, F Perez-Ruiz, N Schlesinger, eds. *Gout*, pp. 164–72. Future Medicine, London.

Dalbeth N and Merriman T (2009). Crystal ball gazing: new therapeutic targets for hyperuricaemia and gout. *Rheumatology*, 48, 222–26.

Dalbeth N and Stamp L (2014). Hyperuricaemia and gout: time for a new staging system? *Annals of the Rheumatic Diseases*, doi: 10.1136/annrheumdis-2014-205304

Dalbeth N, et al. (2010). Cellular characterization of the gouty tophus: a quantitative analysis. *Arthritis & Rheumatism*, 62, 1549–56.

DeBosch B, et al. (2014). Early-onset metabolic syndrome in mice lacking the intestinal uric acid transporter SLC2A9. *Nature Communications*, 5, art. no. 4642.

Dinour D, et al. (2010). Homozygous SLC2A9 mutations cause severe renal hypouricemia. *Journal of the American Society of Nephrology*, 21, 64–72.

Doring A, et al. (2008). SLC2A9 influences uric acid concentrations with pronounced sex-specific effects. *Nature Genetics*, 40, 430–6.

Fuchs TA, et al. (2007). Novel cell death program leads to neutrophil extracellular traps. *Journal of Cell Biology*, 176, 231–41.

Gibson T, et al. (1984). Hyperuricaemia, gout and kidney function in New Zealand Maori men. *British Journal of Rheumatology*, 23, 276–82.

Ichida K, et al. (2012). Decreased extra-renal urate excretion is a common cause of hyperuricemia. *Nature Communications*, 3, art. no. 764.

Jansen TL, et al. (2014). New gout test: enhanced ex vivo cytokine production from PBMCS in common gout patients and a gout patient with Kearns-Sayre syndrome. *Clinical Rheumatology*, 33, 1341–46.

Johnson RJ, et al. (2009). Hypothesis: could excessive fructose intake and uric acid cause type 2 diabetes? *Endocrine Reviews*, 30, 96–116.

Joosten LAB, et al. (2010). Engagement of fatty acids with toll-like receptor 2 drives interleukin-1β production via the ASC/caspase 1 pathway in monosodium urate monohydrate crystal–induced gouty arthritis. *Arthritis & Rheumatism*, 62, 3237–48.

Köttgen A, et al. (2013). Genome-wide association analyses identify 18 new loci associated with serum urate concentrations. *Nature Genetics*, 45, 145–54.

Kratzer JT, et al. (2014). Evolutionary history and metabolic insights of ancient mammalian uricases. *Proceedings of the National Academy of Sciences*, 111, 3763–68.

Liu-Bryan R and Terkeltaub R (2012). Tophus biology and pathogenesis of monosodium urate crystal–induced inflammation. In R Terkeltaub, ed. *Gout and other crystal arthropathies*, pp. 59–71. Elsevier Saunders, Philadelphia.

Liu-Bryan R, et al. (2005). Innate immunity conferred by toll-like receptors 2 and 4 and myeloid differentiation factor 88 expression is pivotal to monosodium urate monohydrate crystal–induced inflammation. *Arthritis and Rheumatism*, 52, 2936–46.

Mandal AK and Mount DB (2015). The molecular physiology of uric acid homeostasis. *Annual Review of Physiology*, 77, 323–45.

Merriman TR and Dalbeth N (2011). The genetic basis of hyperuricaemia and gout. *Joint Bone Spine*, 78, 35–40.

Misawa T, et al. (2013). Microtubule-driven spatial arrangement of mitochondria promotes activation of the NLRP3 inflammasome. *Nature Immunology*, 14, 454–60.

Phipps-Green AJ, et al. (2014). Twenty-eight loci that influence serum urate levels: analysis of association with gout. *Annals of the Rheumatic Diseases*. doi: 10.1136/annrheumdis-2014-205877.

Rasheed H, et al. (2013). Association of the lipoprotein receptor-related protein 2 gene with gout and non-additive interaction with alcohol consumption. *Arthritis Research & Therapy*, 15, R177.

Roch-Ramel F, and Guisan B (1999). Renal transport of urate in humans. *Physiology*, 14, 80–84.

Schauer C, et al. (2014). Aggregated neutrophil extracellular traps limit inflammation by degrading cytokines and chemokines. *Nature Medicine*, 20, 511–17.

Shi Y, Mucsi AD, and Ng G (2010). Monosodium urate crystals in inflammation and immunity. *Immunological Review*, 233, 203–17.

Chapter 3

Epidemiology

Key points

- Owing to the different means of ascertaining prevalence between studies it is difficult to compare prevalence between countries.
- Country-specific studies that collect data with the same methodology show that the prevalence of gout is increasing.
- Factors that influence the prevalence of gout are inherited genetic factors and environmental exposures.
- Some foods that increase serum urate levels and trigger acute gouty arthritis are risk factors - red meat and beer are the best established but seafood and sugar-sweetened beverages also increase serum urate levels and are strong anecdotal triggers of flares.
- Diuretics associate with increased serum urate and the risk of gout.
- Hyperuricaemia and gout are co-morbid with other metabolic conditions, the most prominent being heart and renal disease and type 2 diabetes.
- Collectively the evidence does not suggest that increased serum urate levels are clinically detrimental, except in gout, nephrolithiasis, and perhaps progression of heart and kidney disease.

3.1 Prevalence of gout

Because of different approaches to ascertaining gout—from self-report in surveillance surveys (which depends on inconsistent recall and is prone to errant self-diagnosis) to physician diagnosis (which depends on the patient seeking medical advice) to the use of hospital or clinic records (prone to selection bias)—it is virtually impossible to determine the exact prevalence of gout in individual countries and to compare prevalence between countries. However, changing prevalence can be observed in specific countries using data captured with similar methodologies.

Kuo et al. (2015) present a global review of the prevalence of gout. It highlights an increased prevalence in developed countries but with missing data (mostly from less developed countries) also a feature. In the Global Burden of Disease 2010 report on gout, only two out of 496 data points were from sub-Saharan regions in Africa and only four were from Oceania (Smith et al. 2014). The highest gout prevalence has been reported in populations of Polynesian ancestry in the Oceanic region, which correlates with the observation that these populations have the highest mean serum urate levels worldwide (Figure 3.1) (Gosling et al. 2014). A recent New Zealand study used administrative data to estimate age- and sex-standardized prevalence of gout (Winnard et al. 2012). This study highlights several established features of

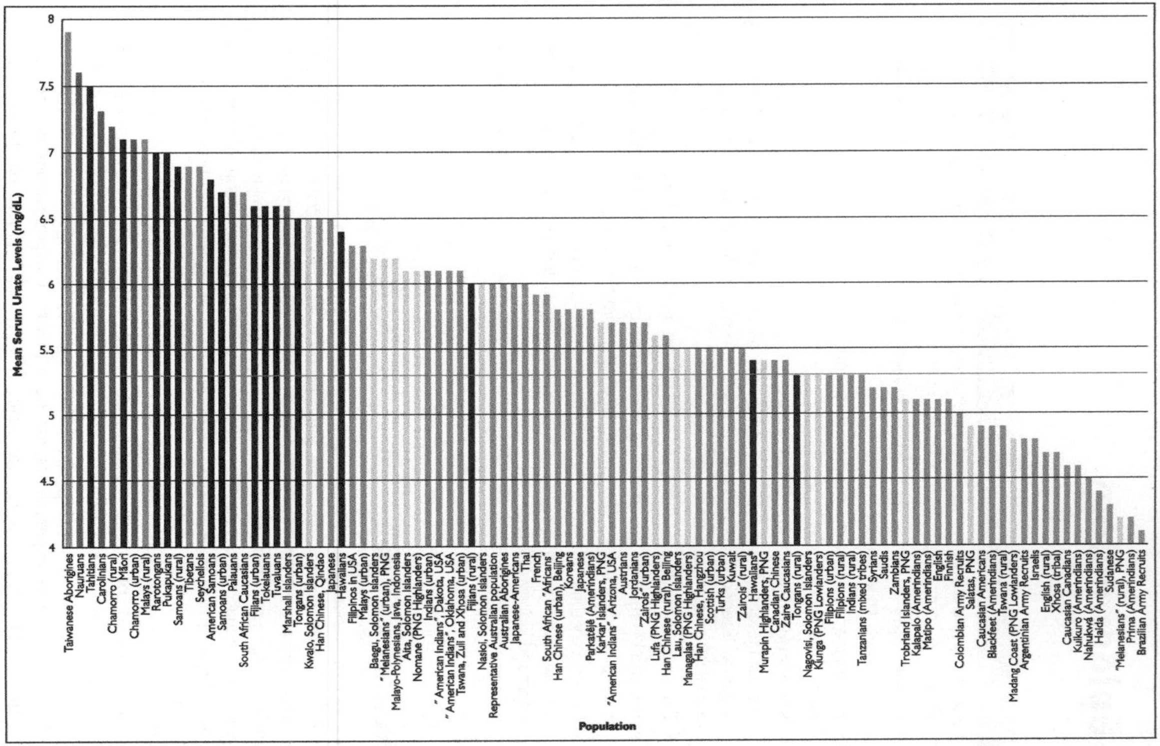

Figure 3.1 Mean serum urate concentrations (measured in mg/dL) worldwide. Dark bars indicate Polynesian populations; green bars, Micronesian; yellow bars, Melanesian; blue bars, non-Pacific. The mean urate level worldwide is 5.5 mg/dL. Taken from Gosling et al. (2014).

Source: Springer and the Rheumatology International, Vol 34, 2014, Hyperuricaemia in the Pacific: why the elevated serum urate levels? Anna L. Gosling, Copyright 2013, with kind permission from Springer Science and Business Media.

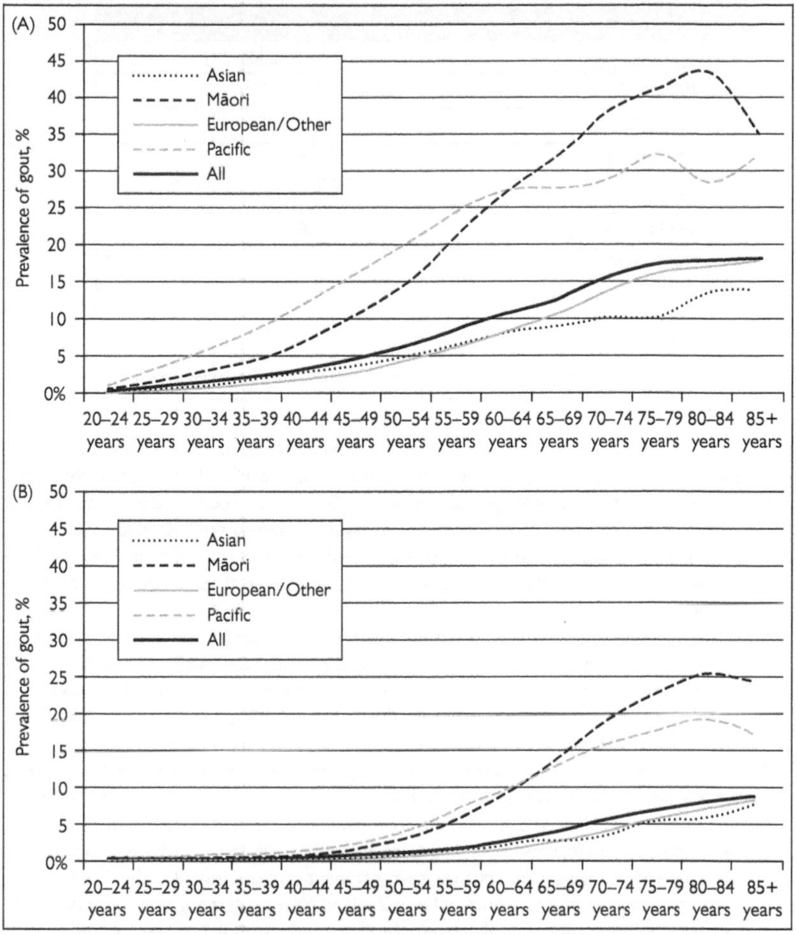

Figure 3.2 Prevalence of gout in the Aotearoa New Zealand Health Tracker population. (A) In men, by age and ethnicity. (B) In women, by age and ethnicity. Taken from Winnard et al. (2012).
Source: Doone Winnard et al, National prevalence of gout derived from administrative health data in Aotearoa New Zealand, Rheumatology, 2012, Vol 51, No. 5, by permission of Oxford University Press.

gout risk factors which are generalizable to other populations and countries (Figure 3.2; see also Kuo et al. 2015).

First, there is variable prevalence between population groups within a single country: in New Zealand, prevalence is 3.2% in Europeans, 6.1% in the native Māori population, and 7.6% in the immigrant Pacific Island population. This is likely due to a combination of increased genetic risk factors for hyperuricaemia and gout, and different environmental conditions, including socioeconomic status. To better understand risk factors for gout, it is important that country-specific prevalence studies analyse separate ethnic groups. Second, there is a marked difference in prevalence between sexes, with a three- to fourfold higher prevalence in men <50 years of age. The sex difference, less pronounced in people >70 years of age, is likely

Table 3.1 Prevalence of gout over time (adults)

Year (country)	Prevalence (%)
1960 (NZ*)	0.3/2.7
1966 (NZ)	0.9/6.0
1990s (UK)	1.4
1997 (NZ)	2.9/6.4
1998 (USA)	2.6
2008 (USA)	3.9
2012 (UK) (Kuo et al. 2014)	3.2
2012 (NZ) (Winnard et al. 2012)	3.2/6.1

*New Zealand studies give the European prevalence (left) and Māori prevalence (right).

related to sex hormones: menopause is associated with increased urate levels, and use of postmenopausal hormone is associated with reduced urate levels. Third, there is increased prevalence with age; for example, prevalence in the 70–74-year group is 10.3%. The sex and age findings are also reflected in the incidence of gout, at least in the UK (Kuo et al. 2014). Finally, prevalence increases with increased social deprivation: in New Zealand those in the most deprived quintile were 41% more likely to have gout than those in the least deprived quintile (Winnard et al. 2012).

Within populations and countries trends in gout prevalence can be identified. Studies using equivalent methodologies from the UK (using a primary health care database) and the United States (self-reported gout in an interviewer-administered survey) suggest that the prevalence of gout has increased by more than one percent from the 1990s to the 2000s (Table 3.1). The New Zealand data in Table 3.1 were collected using different methodologies (the three earlier studies were by physical examination of regionally selected cohorts and the fourth from administrative data); however, it is notable that the prevalence of gout in Europeans has increased markedly since the 1960s, whereas the prevalence in Māori has been stable at ~6%. Collectively, the data summarized in Table 3.1 are consistent with the hypothesis of prevalence being modulated by the impact of a changing environment on a population with a fixed genetic burden, with the levelling of prevalence in New Zealand Māori suggesting that 'saturation' has been reached. This 'saturation' has also been noted in obesity prevalence in some countries.

3.2 Environmental risk factors

Compared to most other complex conditions, environmental risk factors for gout have been relatively easy to identify, with advice regarding some factors now established in most gout management approaches, both clinical and in patient support groups. It is clear from epidemiological and clinical studies that certain foods alter the risk of gout by increasing or decreasing serum urate levels, systematically reviewed by Singh et al. (2011). Based on patient reports, these foods are also widely accepted as triggers of gout attacks. Alcohol and purine-rich foods are proven triggers from case-control crossover studies. However, given the close association of these foods with the triggering of painful attacks of gouty arthritis, there is an argument that avoidance of these foods is given overweighted importance in primary and secondary care.

Four foods are established as associated with increased serum urate levels and increased risk of incident gout: meat (particularly red meat), seafood, alcohol, and sugar-sweetened beverages (SSB). Within the alcohol food group, beer and spirits are consistently associated with increased urate levels and risk of gout, whereas wine is not associated with either (Choi et al. 2004a; Choi and Curhan 2004; Rasheed et al. 2013). Urate is a catabolic product of purine metabolism; therefore purine-rich food groups are often studied. Although increasing intake of purine-rich foods was associated with increased risk of recurrent gout attacks (Zhang et al. 2012), a purine-rich vegetable diet was not associated with increased risk of incident gout (Choi et al. 2004b). The collective evidence therefore suggests that it is characteristics of the individual foods (e.g. red meat, beer) that are important. For example, while the hepatic metabolism of alcohol is known to increase urate levels, and alcohol is known to reduce renal clearance of uric acid, the fact that wine is not associated with urate levels or risk of gout suggests that there are other factors in beer and spirits (e.g. sugar-sweetened mixers in spirits could influence the risk of gout, or wine could contain a gout-protective substance or substances).

Of red meat, seafood, alcohol, and SSB, the latter has the clearest biological mechanism for increasing urate levels. These beverages are predominantly sweetened either with high-fructose corn syrup (HFCS; 55–60% fructose) or sucrose (50% fructose). Unlike glucose, the metabolism of fructose is not subjected to feedback regulation by downstream metabolites, thus fructose ingestion and subsequent metabolism by fructokinase rapidly increases urate production by increasing hepatic ATP degradation to AMP, a urate precursor. Controlled fructose- and SSB-feeding results in a rise in urate levels within 30 minutes (Dalbeth et al. 2013; Le et al. 2012), with HFCS-sweetened beverages having a greater increase than sucrose-sweetened beverages (Le et al. 2012).

Fruit is a natural source of fructose and has been tested for association with gout, with conflicting results. Men from the Health Professionals' Follow-up Study who consumed one apple or one orange per day were shown to have an increased risk for incident gout compared to those who had an apple or orange less than once a month. However, there was no association between total fruit, apples, or oranges and risk of incident gout in women from the Nurses' Health Study, and a smaller study reported that each daily piece of fruit is associated with a reduced risk of incident gout in active men.

Other foods and vitamin C lower urate levels and decrease the risk of gout. The best established are dairy products (Choi et al. 2004b; Choi et al. 2005). A small crossover trial demonstrated both serum urate–lowering and fractional excretion of urate–increasing effects of skim milk, and a single randomized controlled trial has suggested that daily ingestion of skim milk powder can reduce the frequency of gout flares. Cherry consumption protects from recurrent gout attacks in a case-control crossover study, and a small study in women showed a reduction in serum urate levels with daily cherry consumption. There is an inverse correlation between coffee and risk of incident gout in women and men, and ≥6 servings of coffee per day is associated with reduced serum urate levels. The mechanism is unclear and likely to be related to the non-caffeine component of coffee, as decaffeinated coffee also shows a serum urate–lowering and gout-protective effect, and tea consumption shows no association with gout risk or serum urate levels. Vitamin C intake was associated with reduction in serum urate levels in men and reduced the risk of incident gout in men, consistent with the effect of a randomized controlled trial of the effect of vitamin C on serum urate levels. Vitamin C may reduce the risk of gout by increasing renal excretion of uric acid.

Diuretic medication (both loop and thaizide diuretics) has long been established to be associated with urate levels and the risk of gout in observational studies (Gibson 2013; Singh et al. 2011). However, the biological mechanism(s) remains elusive, with extremely few mechanistic studies addressing this clinically important question. One in-vitro experiment showed that the NPT4 renal uric acid transporter exhibited allele-specific interaction with bumetanide and furosemide. Interestingly, one observational study found no association between diuretic use and risk of gout after adjustment for hypertension, heart failure, and myocardial infarction (Janssens et al. 2006). This raises the possibility that the studies reporting association between diuretics and hyperuricaemia and gout could be confounded by the co-morbid association between gout and these conditions (see Section 3.3), which are the main indicators for diuretic use.

3.3 Co-morbidity: is urate causal of other metabolic conditions?

Gout is more than an arthritic joint, being co-morbid with a number of other prominent metabolic conditions: cardiovascular disease, type 2 diabetes, hypertension, renal failure, and dyslipidemia. The observational associations between gout/hyperuricaemia and these conditions will not be reiterated here, as they are established in the literature and reviewed in detail elsewhere (Robinson and Horsburgh 2014; Roddy and Choi 2014). They are all clinically relevant risk factors for hyperuricaemia and gout. However the causal relationship (if any) between hyperuricaemia/gout and these conditions is unclear.

A central question in the association between gout and cardiovascular disease (CVD), for example, is whether gout is causal of CVD, CVD is causal of gout, or do specific features of each disease promote the other? For example, does urate cause endothelial damage in CVD, and/or does systemic inflammation in CVD increase the risk of gout? Alternatively, the observational relationship could be based on unmeasured causal factors (e.g. environmental exposure) that independently cause both gout and co-morbidities.

One approach that can shed light on the causal relationships is a genetic epidemiology technique called Mendelian randomization. This technique can be likened to a randomized clinical trial, whereby individuals are randomly assigned to separate exposure (allele that raises biological exposure of interest, e.g. urate) and control (other allele) groups at gamete formation and conception, and followed for disease outcome. Provided the groups are equally exposed to the same environment, then the genetic variants can be used as 'instruments'—not generally susceptible to the confounding of traditional associative studies—to test that the biological exposure they regulate is associated with and causal of disease. This approach has been applied to serum urate, with no evidence that urate is causal of CVD, reduced renal function, hypertension, type 2 diabetes, or dyslipidemia. There is evidence for reverse causality, in that body mass index and dyslipidemia are causal of increased urate level. While any support by Mendelian randomization for hyperuricaemia being causal of the development of the co-morbid conditions is scant, there is, however, evidence—also from Mendelian randomization studies—that hyperuricaemia can contribute to progression of CVD and renal disease.

One other approach for investigating the possible causal role for urate in co-morbid conditions is to evaluate outcomes in clinical trials with the use of urate-lowering therapy. In the control of essential hypertension in adolescents, the use of allopurinol reduces blood pressure. There is evidence that allopurinol can improve outcomes in chronic kidney and heart disease, and can reduce left ventricular mass in ischaemic heart disease, although larger trials are needed to confirm these observations. However, the administration of allopurinol benefits endothelial function by reducing vascular oxidative stress via inhibition of the reactive oxygen species- and urate-producing xanthine oxidase, rather than by the lowering of urate (George et al. 2006; Rajendra et al. 2011). Finally, a Mendelian randomization study shows that increased serum levels are causal of *improved* renal function in men with the *activity* of renal uric acid transporter(s) in raising urate levels possibly improving renal function (Hughes et al. 2014).

3.4 Conclusion

There is much research to be done in understanding the relationship between hyperuricaemia and other metabolic conditions. Understanding the various biological mechanisms should improve management of gout in the presence of co-morbidities. Collectively the evidence does not suggest that increased serum urate levels are clinically detrimental, except in gout, nephrolithiasis, and perhaps progression of heart and kidney disease. Given the increasing observational epidemiological evidence for a protective role of urate in neurological disease and dementia—including an inosine (urate purine precursor) dosing trial that improved outcome in Parkinson's disease (Schwarzschild et al. 2014)—the application of urate lowering outside of gout and other specific clinical settings should be carefully considered.

References

Choi, HK and Curhan G (2004). Beer, liquor, and wine consumption and serum uric acid level: the Third National Health and Nutrition Examination Survey. *Arthritis Care & Research, 51*, 1023–9.

Choi HK, et al. (2004a). Alcohol intake and risk of incident gout in men: a prospective study. *Lancet*, 363, 1277–81.

Choi HK, et al. (2004b). Purine-rich foods, dairy and protein intake, and the risk of gout in men. *New England Journal of Medicine*, 350, 1093–103.

Choi HK, Liu S, Curhan G (2005). Intake of purine-rich foods, protein, and dairy products and relationship to serum levels of uric acid: The Third National Health and Nutrition Examination Survey. *Arthritis & Rheumatism*, 52, 283–9.

Dalbeth N, et al. (2013). Population-specific influence of SLC2A9 genotype on the acute hyperuricaemic response to a fructose load. *Annals of the Rheumatic Diseases*, 72, 1868–73.

George J, et al. (2006). High-dose allopurinol improves endothelial function by profoundly reducing vascular oxidative stress and not by lowering uric acid. *Circulation*, 114, 2508–16.

Gibson TJ (2013). Hypertension, its treatment, hyperuricaemia and gout. *Current Opinion in Rheumatology*, 25, 217–22.

Gosling AL, Matisoo-Smith E, and Merriman TR (2014). Hyperuricaemia in the Pacific: why the elevated serum urate levels? *Rheumatology International*, 34, 743–57.

Hughes K, et al. (2014). Mendelian randomization analysis associates increased serum urate, due to genetic variation in uric acid transporters, with improved renal function. *Kidney International*, 85, 344–51.

Janssens HJ, et al. (2006). Gout, not induced by diuretics? a case-control study from primary care. *Annals of the Rheumatic Diseases*, 65, 1080–83.

Kuo C-F, et al. (2014). Rising burden of gout in the UK but continuing suboptimal management: a nationwide population study. *Annals of the Rheumatic Diseases*, 74, 661–67.

Kuo C-F, et al. (2015). Global epidemiology of gout: prevalence, incidence and risk factors. *Nature Reviews Rheumatology*. doi:10.1038/nrrheum.2015.91

Le MT, et al. (2012). Effects of high-fructose corn syrup and sucrose on the pharmacokinetics of fructose and acute metabolic and hemodynamic responses in healthy subjects. *Metabolism*, 61, 641–51.

Rajendra NS, et al. (2011). Mechanistic insights into the therapeutic use of high-dose allopurinol in angina pectoris. *Journal of the American College of Cardiology*, 58, 820–28.

Rasheed H, et al. (2013). Association of the lipoprotein receptor-related protein 2 gene with gout and non-additive interaction with alcohol consumption. *Arthritis Research & Therapy*, 15, R177.

Robinson PC and Horsburgh S (2014). Gout: Joints and beyond, epidemiology, clinical features, treatment and co-morbidities. *Maturitas*, 78, 245–51.

Roddy E and Choi HK (2014). Epidemiology of gout. *Rheumatic Disease Clinics of North America*, 40, 155–75.

Schwarzschild MA, et al. (2014). Inosine to increase serum and cerebrospinal fluid urate in Parkinson disease: a randomized clinical trial. *JAMA Neurology*, 71, 141–50.

Singh JA, Reddy SG, and Kundukulam J (2011). Risk factors for gout and prevention: a systematic review of the literature. *Current Opinion in Rheumatology*, 23, 192–202.

Smith E, et al. (2014). The global burden of gout: estimates from the Global Burden of Disease 2010 study. Annals of the Rheumatic Diseases, 73, 1470–76.

Winnard D, et al. (2012). National prevalence of gout derived from administrative health data in Aotearoa New Zealand. Rheumatology (Oxford, England), 51, 901–9.

Zhang Y, et al. (2012). Purine-rich foods intake and recurrent gout attacks. Annals of the Rheumatic Diseases, 71, 1448–53.

Chapter 4

Genetic basis of hyperuricaemia and gout

Key points

- About 60% of the variance in serum urate levels can be explained by inherited genetic factors, but the extent of the contribution of genetic factors to gout in the presence of hyperuricaemia is not known.
- Genome-wide association studies in Europeans have identified 28 loci controlling serum urate levels, although the molecular basis of the majority of these genetic associations is currently unknown.
- The *SLC2A9* and *ABCG2* renal and gut uric acid transporters have very strong effects on urate levels and the risk of gout.
- Other uric acid transporters (e.g. *SLC22A11/OAT4, SLC22A12/URAT1*) and a glycolysis gene (*GCKR*) are associated with urate levels.
- Environmental exposures such as sugar-sweetened beverages and alcohol interact with urate-associated genetic variants in an unpredictable fashion.
- Very little is known about the genetic control of gout in the presence of hyperuricaemia, formation of monosodium urate (MSU) crystals, and the immune response.

As outlined in Chapter 2, there are a number of key checkpoints in the development of acute gouty arthritis: hyperuricaemia, crystal deposition, and the subsequent inflammatory response. At each of these points, inherited genetic variants—both common variants of weak effect and rare variants of stronger effect—will collectively explain a proportion of the variance in phenotype. Or, put more simply, they will explain why some people are, for example, hyperuricaemic and some are not. This chapter will review the genetic basis of hyperuricaemia and gout, including an emphasis on new understanding of the aetiology of gout that genetic approaches have revealed. The focus will be on common gout, with rare monogenic causes of gout briefly discussed.

4.1 Heritability of urate and gout

Population variance in most disease phenotypes is governed by inherited genetic variation, environmental exposures, and the interaction between the two. Heritability is defined as the proportion of phenotypic variability that is explained by inherited genetic variants in a defined population in a defined environment. In humans it is usually calculated from twin studies that compare phenotypic concordance between mono- and dizygotic twin pairs, and is called the 'broad-sense' heritability (H^2). It includes all genetic effects including epistasis (nonadditive genetic interactions) and nonadditive interactions with environmental exposures. Most human complex phenotypes have heritability estimates of greater than 50%. This includes serum urate levels and renal clearance of uric acid, both with an estimated heritability of ~60%. A Taiwanese study using health insurance records from the entire population reported a heritable component for gout of 35% in men and 17% in women (Kuo et al. 2015). A United States study on 512 male twins pairs reported no significant heritability for gout (Krishnan et al. 2012); paradoxically, this study reported significant heritability for hyperuricaemia. Thus there is a clear heritable component to serum urate levels even though heritability estimates for gout are very unclear, particularly when considering the possible genetic control of MSU crystal formation and innate immune response.

4.2 Genome-wide scanning for genetic variants associated with serum urate levels

A genome-wide association study scans the genome, in an unbiased fashion using common genetic variants (typically single nucleotide polymorphisms), for loci causally associated with a particular phenotype. This approach typically does not detect uncommon (<5%) genetic variants associated with phenotype, and the common genetic variants that are detected typically explain only a very small proportion of variance in phenotype (although the *SLC2A9* and *ABCG2* loci in urate control are very relevant exceptions in explaining relatively large proportions of variance in urate). Genes contained within the associated loci are candidates for involvement in causal pathogenic pathways. The genome-wide studies have to include a large number of participants in order to be able to detect genome-wide statistical significance at very low *P* values (usually $<10^{-8}$) that are required in order to account for the inherent simultaneous multiple testing of millions of genetic variants.

In a genome-wide association study (GWAS) of >140,000 Europeans, Köttgen et al. (2013) reported statistically significant associations of 28 separate genetic loci with serum urate levels. This study confirmed the association with urate levels of ten loci discovered in earlier and smaller GWA studies. Reviewed elsewhere (Merriman et al. 2013), the ten are dominated by loci containing genes that were either known (*SLC22A11/OAT4, SLC22A12/URAT1, SLC17A1/NPT1, PDZK1*) or novel (*SLC2A9/GLUT9, ABCG2*) renal and gut transporters of uric acid. The *GCKR* (glucokinase regulatory protein) locus implicates production of urate by glycolysis, with the functional relevance of the remaining loci (*SLC16A9/MCT9, INHBC, RREB1*) unclear, although *MCT9* may be a renal sodium transporter and has been linked to urate via carnitine metabolism. Predictably, most, but not all, of these ten loci consistently associate with gout in multiple ancestral groups (Köttgen et al. 2013; Phipps-Green et al. 2014; Urano et al. 2013).

The lead associated genetic variants at *SLC2A9* and *ABCG2* collectively explain, depending on sex, 3–4% of the variance in urate levels. On average, the urate-raising allele at *SLC2A9* increases serum urate by 0.373 mg/dL (0.022 mmol/L) and the urate-raising allele at *ABCG2* by 0.217 mg/dL (0.013 mmol/L) (Köttgen et al. 2013)—both clinically significant amounts. *SLC2A9* and *ABCG2* have equivalent effects in men, with *SLC2A9* a stronger effect in women than men, and vice versa for *ABCG2* (Köttgen et al. 2013). Sex-specific effects aside, both loci (in particular *SLC2A9*) exert extremely strong control on urate levels, when compared to the effect of the other 26 confirmed urate loci that collectively explain a similar proportion of variance. Thus there is considerable research interest in the molecular basis of urate control by *SLC2A9* and *ABCG2*, and their clinical significance.

4.3 Genetic complexity at *SLC2A9*

The urate association signal at the *SLC2A9* locus is extensive, with hundreds of genetic variants extremely strongly associated. The strongest association encompasses a very large region

(500 kb) with the single nucleotide polymorphism rs12498742 the most strongly associated (Köttgen et al. 2013). It is thus difficult to determine whether the genetic effect at *SLC2A9* is caused by a single genetic variant with very strong effect that drives the widespread association owing to extensive intermarker 'linkage disequilibrium'. This can be studied by 'conditional analysis', whereby the association with phenotype of other variants at a locus is tested conditional on the effect of the strongest associated variant at the locus. Conditional analysis suggests multiple independent genetic effects at *SLC2A9*. GWA studies of serum urate levels in East Asians and African Americans also reveal the strongest genome-wide association with urate at *SLC2A9* (Charles et al. 2011; Okada et al. 2012), but with a different single nucleotide polymorphism (SNP) variant (rs3775948). Interestingly, this is the second-strongest independent signal in the Köttgen et al. (2013) European study. This suggests that there are at least two causal variants controlling urate levels at *SLC2A9* that operate in Europeans, with only one operating in East Asians. The most strongly associated European variant was not detected as a genetic controller of urate levels in East Asians because of the rarity of the minor allele.

It is possible that the causative serum urate–raising variant in Europeans (marked by Köttgen et al. [2013] rs12498742 SNP) increases the expression levels of an *SLC2A9* isoform (*SLC2A9b* [GLUT9S]), with a 28 residue portion missing from the N-terminus that is predominantly expressed on the apical (urine) membrane, presumably increasing reabsorption of uric acid from the filtered urine.

4.4 *ABCG2*

Association of the *ABCG2* locus with serum urate was first reported in the GWAS of Dehghan et al. (2008). The genetic basis is considerably simpler than that at *SLC2A9*, with the association signal reported as being driven solely by *rs2231142* (Q141K); the variant is highly likely to be causal (Woodward et al. 2013). The ABCG2 protein (also known as breast cancer resistance protein) is a multidrug transport protein transporting a wide range of molecules, including chemotherapeutic agents. It is a secretory uric acid transporter in the proximal tubule and the gut, with the mechanistic impact of the urate-increasing 141K allele reviewed in Chapter 2. Histone deacetylase inhibitors are able to correct the ABCG2 141K urate-increasing 'defect' (Woodward et al. 2013) by relocalizing the misfolded form of ABCG2 141K to the cell surface (Basseville et al. 2012). Of clinical relevance, a GWAS for genetic variants influencing the urate-lowering response to the xanthine oxidase inhibitor allopurinol identified the *ABCG2* 141K allele to associate with reduced response at a stringent genome-wide level of significance (Wen et al. 2015), even after accounting for baseline serum urate levels. While this pharmacogenomic finding requires replication in a data set where compliance with allopurinol treatment is verified by measuring the active metabolite oxypurinol, it raises the possibility of *ABCG2* genotype being used to predict allopurinol response and perhaps increase dose in individuals with the 141K allele.

4.5 The Köttgen et al. (2013) GWAS in serum urate levels

The large GWAS conducted by Köttgen et al. (2013) reported 18 new loci with a weaker effect on urate levels than the previously identified ten, with the new 18 explaining a further 1.8% of variance in urate levels compared to 5.2% for the ten previously known loci. Notably, none of the new loci contained genes encoding known uric acid transporters, although an association that was almost genome-wide significant was detected in the *SLC2A7* locus (encoding the organic anion transporter 2) in a candidate gene secondary analysis. Summarized in Table 4.1, the Köttgen et al. study contains a treasure trove of information on the control of urate levels.

Table 4.1 Summary of the 28 genome-wide significant urate loci detected by Köttgen et al. (2013)

	GRAIL gene	Effect size (male/female[1]) (mg/dL)	FEUA (Y/N)[2]	Association signal	Probable causal gene[3]	Strongest candidate(s)[4,5]
Old loci						
rs1471633	*PDZK1*	0.059	N	Within *PDZK1*	*PDZK1*	-
rs1260326	*GCKR*	0.074 (0.091/0.063)	Y	Spans >20 genes	-	*GCKR*
rs12498742	*SLC2A9*	0.373 (0.269/0.460)	Y	Spans 4 genes	*SLC2A9*	-
rs2231142	*ABCG2*	0.217 (0.280/0.181)	Y	Spans 4 genes	*ABCG2*	-
rs675209	*RREB1*	0.061	Y	Upstream and within *RREB1*	-	*RREB1*
rs1165151	*SLC17A3*	0.091	N	Spans 20 genes	-	*SLC17A1-A4*
rs1171614	*SLC16A9*	0.079	N	Spans 2 genes	-	-
rs2078267	*SLC22A11*	0.073	Y	Within *SLC22A11*	*SLC22A11*	-
rs478607	*SLC22A12*	0.047	Y	Spans 6 genes	-	*SLC22A12*
rs3741414	*INHBC*	0.072 (0.091/0.057)	N	Spans 7 genes	-	-
New loci						
rs11264341	*PKLR*	0.050	N	Spans 2 genes	-	-
rs17050272	*INHBB*	0.035	N	Intergenic	*INHBB*	-
rs2307384	*ACVR2A*	0.029	N	Spans 3 genes	-	-
rs6770152	*MUSTN1*	0.044	N	Spans 3 genes	-	-
rs17632159	*TMEM171*	0.039	N	Intergenic	-	-
rs729761	*VEGFA*	0.047	N	Intergenic	-	-
rs1178977	*MLXIPL*	0.047	N	Spans 5 genes	-	*MLXIPL*
rs10480300	*PRKAG2*	0.035	N	Within *PRKAG2*	-	*PRKAG2*

rs17786744	*STC1*	0.029	N	Intergenic	-	-
rs2941484	*HNF4G*	0.044	N	Within *HNF4G*		*HNF4G*
rs10821905	*ASAH2*	0.057	N	Within *A1CF*		*A1CF*
rs642803	*LTBP3*	0.036	N	Spans 6 genes	-	-
rs653178	*PTPN11*[6]	0.035	N	Spans 3 genes	-	-
rs1394125	*NRG4*	0.043 (0.061/0.032)	Y	Spans 4 genes	-	-
rs6598541	*IGF1R*	0.043	Y	Within *IGFR1*	-	*IGFR1*
rs7193778	*NFAT5*	0.046	Y	Intergenic	-	-
rs7188445	*MAF*	0.032	N	Intergenic	-	-
rs7224610	*HLF*	0.042	Y	Within *HLF*	-	*HLF*
rs2079742	*C17ORF82*	0.043	N	Downstream and within *BCAS3*	-	-
rs164009	*PRPSAP1*	0.028	N	Within QRICH2	-	-

Source: Taken from Merriman (2015).

[1] Male and female effect sizes are given for loci where there was a significant sex-specific difference.

[2] Fractional excretion of uric acid (FEUA) was tested by Köttgen et al. on a considerably smaller subset (n = 6799), meaning that inadequate power may contribute to lack of association seen at loci of weaker effect.

[3] A probable causal gene either has very strong functional evidence (*SLC2A9, ABCG2*), strong functional evidence combined with association signal restricted to the gene (*PDZK1*, *SLC22A11*), or very strong eSNP evidence (*INHBB*).

[4] A 'strongest candidate' is listed when the locus contains a candidate with strong functional evidence (*GCKR, SLC17A1-A4, SLC22A12*), has the association signal tightly restricted to the named gene, or has strong eSNP evidence (*MLXIPL*).

[5] RREB1: ras responsive element (zinc-finger) binding protein, has been genetically implicated in type 2 diabetes associated end-stage kidney disease; PRKAG2: protein kinase, AMP-activated, gamma 2 non-catalytic subunit, has been genetically implicated in blood pressure control; HNF4G: hepatocyte nuclear factor 4G, has been genetically implicated in obesity; A1CF: rAPOBEC1 (APOB mRNA editing enzyme) complementation factor; IGFR1: insulin-like growth factor 1 receptor; HLF: hepatic leukemia factor; MLXIPL: carbohydrate element-responsive binding protein; this locus has been identified as a pleiotropic gene for metabolic syndrome and inflammation.

[6] *PTPN11* is ~1 Mb downstream of the association signal and does not harbour any association signal.

Candidate genes at each locus were identified by Köttgen et al. (2013) using 'GRAIL'—a bioinformatic approach that looks for commonalities between associated SNPs, the literature, and published GWA studies. The GRAIL genes were mapped into two broad pathways: glycolysis and inhibins/activins. The relevance of the glycolysis genes to urate likely reflects hepatic production of urate (from sugar and alcohol) via increased generation of glucose-6-phosphate that flows through the pentose-phosphate pathway generating ribose-5-phosphate, a precursor of purine synthesis. Generation of lactic acid from anaerobic glycolysis could also interfere with renal uric acid excretion. This possibility is consistent with the strong association of the *GCKR* locus with fractional excretion of uric acid (the GCKR protein inhibits glucokinase that produces glucose-6-phosphate) (Köttgen et al. 2013). Köttgen et al. noted that the associations with loci containing genes involved in glucose homeostasis fits with the observation that drugs that decrease insulin resistance (e.g. metformin) also tend to decrease serum urate levels, indicating possible new approaches for management of urate levels. The relevance of the inhibins/activins is not clear—Köttgen et al. suggested processes such as energy balance, insulin release, apoptosis, inflammation, and sex hormone regulation.

There is one very important caveat in interpreting the GWAS findings: the considerable majority of the GRAIL-identified genes cannot be assumed as causal. Extensive linkage disequilibrium (intermarker correlation) results in association signals extending for some distance across many loci. Multiple candidate genes can exist (see examples in Figure 4.1), meaning that the gene named by investigators at a particular locus can certainly not be regarded as causal prior to follow-up genetic and functional analyses. One approach employed by Köttgen et al. (2013) to identify likely candidate genes is underpinned by the hypothesis that the causal variant is an 'eSNP' (expression SNP) that influences the expression of the causal gene at the locus. This is a strong hypothesis given that ~70% of genetic variants for common phenotypes identified by GWAS map to regulatory regions of the genome. Köttgen et al. associated the significant SNPs with expression of genes in tissues from publically available databases. The tissues included white blood cells, adipose, various neural cells, fibroblasts, osteoblasts, and liver, although no renal tissue or cell line was analyzed. Of the total 28 genome-wide significant loci, eight showed strong ($P<1\times10^{-4}$) evidence for association with multiple expression probes.

Notable in this analysis was clear evidence that the intergenic association signal at the *INHBB* locus (Figure 4.1) was associated with expression of *INHBB* in the liver. This provides evidence that *INHBB* is the causal gene at this locus. At *ABCG2*, the causal rs2231142 variant (Q141K) was associated with *ABCG2* expression in the liver (Köttgen et al. 2013). There was association with expression of both *BAZ1B* and *MLXIPL* in adipose tissue at the *BAZ1B* locus. This may reflect coordinated expression of closely linked genes, but is consistent with the role of *MLXIPL* (which encodes the glucose-responsive transcription factor ChREBP) in transcriptional activation of glycolytic genes. The eSNP approach does, however, need to be reapplied to the 28 urate loci using a wider range of tissue expression data sets that include renal tissue and gut enteroctyes from different developmental stages.

4.6 **Nonadditive gene-environment interactions in urate and gout control**

A nonadditive interaction is where two factors interact in an unpredictable, nonadditive way. One established interaction in rheumatology is that between smoking and *HLA-DRB1* genotype in determining the risk of anti-citrullinated peptide antibody positive rheumatoid arthritis. In this case the risks of smoking and the *HLA-DRB1* shared epitope multiply (rather than add) in determining the risk of rheumatoid arthritis (RA). These interactions provide knowledge on disease mechanism (the RA example has shed light on the role of smoking in citrullinating

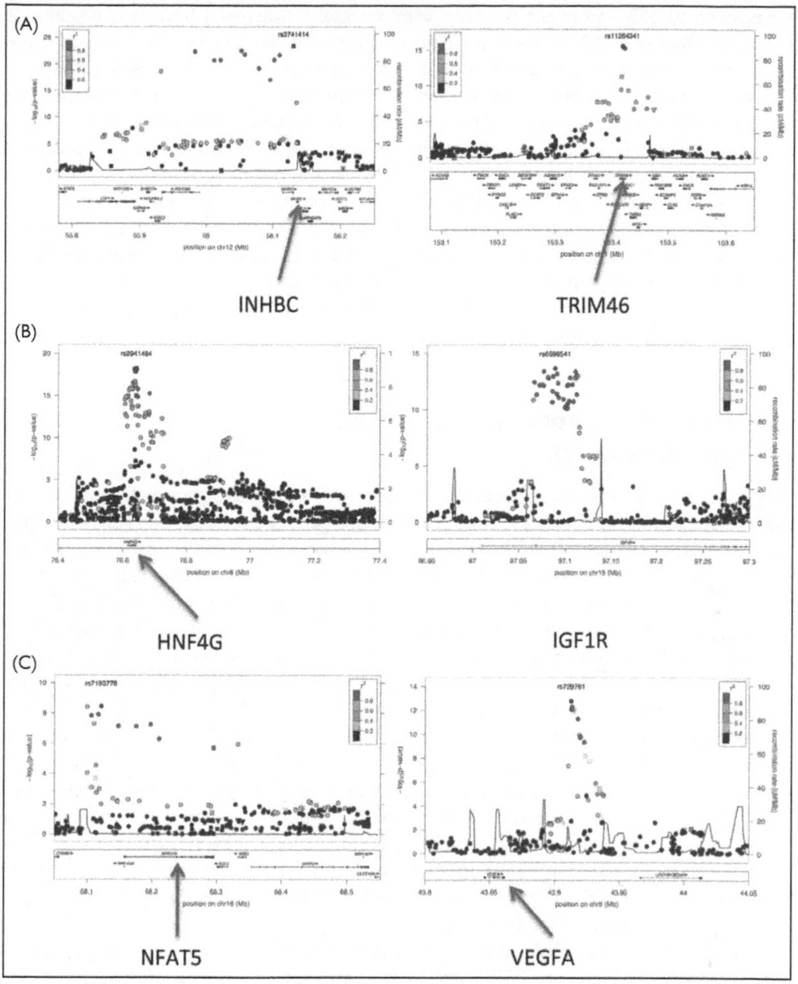

Figure 4.1 LocusZoom pictures of regional association in Europeans. The top associated SNP is labelled, with other associated SNPs coloured according to strength of linkage disequilibrium (correlation). $-\log_{10}P$ is on the left-hand y-axis. Panel A. Illustrating multiple genes underlying a serum urate association signal at the *INHBC* and *TRIM46* loci. Panel B. Examples of association signals that define a single causal gene of high prior probability. Panel C. Examples of intergenic association signals.

peptides in the lung which then stimulate a specific adaptive immune response) and provide possibilities for genotype-specific clinical and public health interventions.

It is established that sugar-sweetened beverages (SSB) increase serum urate levels and increase the risk of gout (see Chapter 3). In an epidemiological study on *SLC2A9*, upon exposure to SSB, the normally urate-lowering allele has a transmutation of effect and *raises* urate in response to SSB—an effect not seen with artificially sweetened beverages (Figure 4.2, top panel) (Batt et al. 2014). From the current state of knowledge, and given the complexity of urate transport in the renal tubule, it is difficult to propose a plausible mechanism to explain this nonadditive interaction. The effects of chronic exposure to fructose-containing SSB may involve other mechanisms (e.g. epigenetic) that influence the expression and activity of SLC2A9. There is nonadditive interaction between alcohol exposure and the lipoprotein receptor–related protein 2 gene (*LRP2 rs2544390*) in the risk of gout in the New Zealand Polynesian (Māori and Pacific) population, where the protective effect of the T-negative genotype is negated by exposure to alcohol (Figure 4.2, bottom panel) (Rasheed et al. 2013). Finally a nonadditive interaction between diuretic use and genotype at each of *SLC2A9* and *SLC22A11* in the risk of incident gout in hypertensive people has been reported in the Atherosclerosis Risk in Communities study (McAdams-DeMarco et al. 2013), although these interactions were not replicated in a larger study (Bao et al. 2015).

4.7 Genetics of gout in the presence of hyperuricaemia

Currently there is only one replicated association of an immune gene with gout: a SNP (rs2149356) within the candidate *TLR4* innate immune gene is associated with gout in Chinese (OR = 1.42, $p < 1\times10^{-4}$) (Qing et al. 2013). This association was not evident in Europeans using unstratified controls (OR = 1.26, p = 0.10) (Merriman et al. unpublished). Importantly, however, the effect size increases considerably and the association is statistically significant when asymptomatic European hyperuricaemic controls are used (OR = 1.63, p = 0.009). If this SNP is further replicated, it—or the causal genetic variant it marks—would probably influence expression of *TLR4* given its intronic location and lack of obvious linkage disequilibrium (correlation) with any non-synonymous variants.

Progress in GWAS in gout has considerably lagged behind that in urate and also in comparison to other equivalent arthropathies (e.g. the latest GWAS on RA analyzed 30,000 cases). The largest gout GWAS in Europeans published to date used 3000 European cases nested within the cohorts used in the Köttgen et al. (2013) urate GWAS, and yielded disappointing results: only *SLC2A9* and *ABCG2* associated at a genome-wide level of significance. A major reason for this is the phenotyping, where cases were ascertained by self-report and/or the use of allopurinol (which is also used in asymptomatic hyperuricaemia), resulting in a 'case' sample set that will include participants without gout.

More recently, smaller GWA studies for gout in Japanese and Chinese sample sets have been published. The Japanese GWAS of 945 male cases and 1213 normouricaemic male controls (Matsuo et al. 2015) identified *SLC2A9* and *ABCG2* as the strongest effects, and also the same effect in *GCKR* as previously identified in gout in other populations (Köttgen et al. 2013; Phipps-Green et al. 2014; Urano et al. 2013). Genome-wide significant signals (after replication) were also observed at the *MYL2-CUX2* and *CNIH-2* loci, pinpointing them as novel gout loci. However, it has not yet been determined whether these loci control hyperuricaemia or aspects of the pathogenic process leading to gout in the presence of hyperuricaemia.

The Chinese GWAS (Li et al. 2015) scanned 1255 male cases and 1848 male controls, with *ABCG2* the strongest genome-wide effect. After replication, there were three genome-wide significant novel loci: *BCAS3*, *RFX3*, and *KCNQ1*. The *BCAS3* signal is at the same locus as one of the European loci identified as associated with urate levels by Köttgen et al. (2013), but genetically independent of the European signal. Again it is not possible to determine whether these loci control acute gouty arthritis in the presence of hyperuricaemia; however, the study design also used asymptomatic hyperuricaemic controls thus increasing the chance of detecting non-urate-controlling loci.

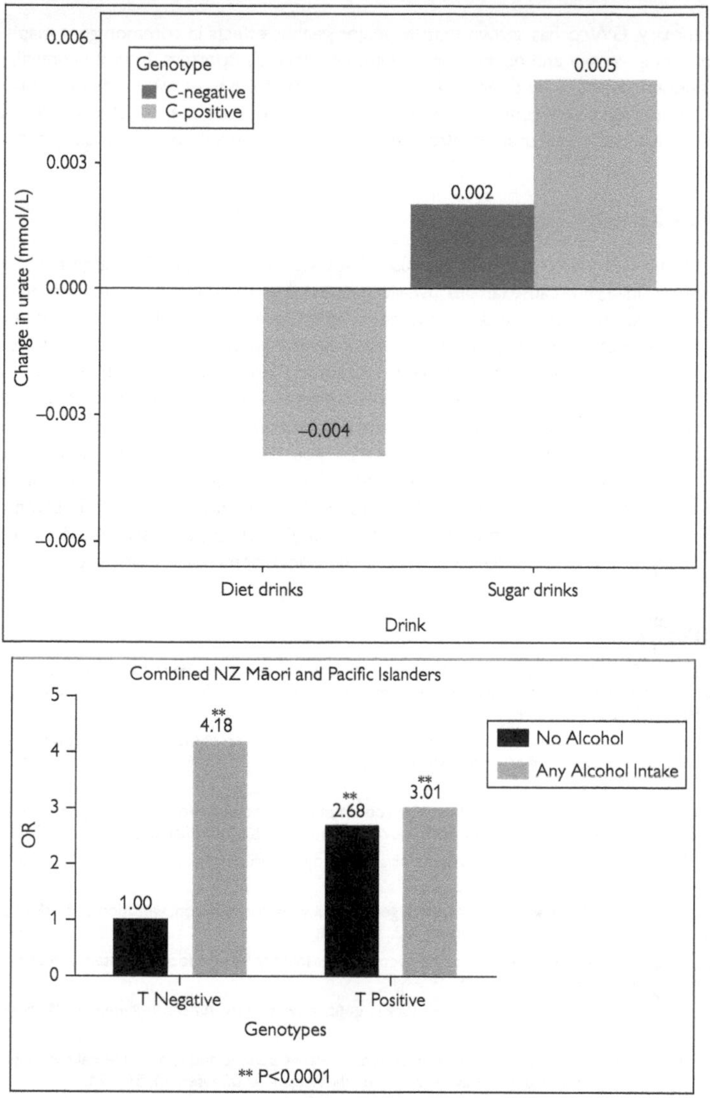

Figure 4.2 Top panel. The nonadditive interaction of SSB consumption with *SLC2A9* genotype in influence of urate levels in Europeans in the Atherosclerosis Risk in Communities data set (Batt et al. 2014). Exposure to artificially sweetened beverages (diet drinks) does not influence the urate-lowering effect of the C-positive genotypes; however, exposure to SSBs reverses the urate-lowering effect of the C-positive genotype. The C-negative diet drinks group is the reference set to 0.000 change in urate. The y-axis corresponds to change in urate per consumption category as defined by Batt et al. (2014). Bottom panel. The nonadditive interaction of alcohol exposure with *LRP2* genotype in risk of gout in New Zealand Polynesians. Any alcohol exposure negates the protective effect of the T-negative genotype at *LRP2 rs2544390*.

Source data (top panel) from Batt, C., et al. (2014), 'Sugar-sweetened beverage consumption: a risk factor for prevalent gout with SLC2A9 genotype-specific effects on serum urate and risk of gout', Ann Rheum Dis, 73, 2101–06.

Source data (bottom panel) from Rasheed, H., et al. (2013), 'Association of the lipoprotein receptor-related protein 2 gene with gout and non-additive interaction with alcohol consumption', Arthritis Res Ther, 15, R177.

In summary, GWAS has shown that the major genetic effects in common gout map within loci containing known and novel renal and gut uric acid transporters. In urate control, there is considerable work to be done in determining its molecular basis within the loci without an obvious candidate causal gene—although glycolysis is implicated as a causal pathway. In acute gouty arthritis, outside of urate control, GWAS has not identified obvious causal genes.

4.8 Rare monogenic gout

Several genes with rare mutant alleles cause clinically distinct forms of familial gout. Mutations in the uromodulin gene cause familial juvenile hyperuricaemic nephropathy, a disease characterized by juvenile onset of hyperuricaemia, gout, and progressive renal failure. Mutations in the signal sequence of the renin gene result in early-onset hyperuricaemia and progressive renal failure by altering the intrarenal angiotensin system and kidney structure. The relatively common *A150P* (*rs1800546*) mutation in the aldolase B gene (*ALDOB*) causes the recessive disease hereditary fructose intolerance (HFI) in approximately two-thirds of European cases; many HFI patients also present with hyperuricaemia and gout. A deficiency in hypoxanthine-guanine phosphoribosyltransferase (HPRT) activity leads to overproduction of urate; mutations in this enzyme result in gout and neurological symptoms (Lesch-Nyhan syndrome). In some cases, mutations in the X-chromosome gene phosphoribosylpyrophosphate synthetase can lead to superactivity, urate overproduction, gout, and neurodevelopmental impairment.

References

Bao Y, et al. (2015). Lack of gene–diuretic interactions on the risk of incident gout: The Nurses' Health Study and Health Professionals Follow-up Study. *Annals of the Rheumatic Diseases*. doi: 10.1136/annrheumdis-2014-206534

Basseville A, et al. (2012). Histone deacetylase inhibitors influence chemotherapy transport by modulating expression and trafficking of a common polymorphic variant of the ABCG2 efflux transporter. *Cancer Research*, 72, 3642–51.

Batt C, et al. (2014). Sugar-sweetened beverage consumption: a risk factor for prevalent gout with SLC2A9 genotype-specific effects on serum urate and risk of gout. *Annals of the Rheumatic Diseases*, 73, 2101–06.

Charles BA, et al. (2011). A genome-wide association study of serum uric acid in African Americans. *BMC Medical Genomics*, 4, 17.

Dehghan A, et al. (2008). Association of three genetic loci with uric acid concentration and risk of gout: a genome-wide association study. *Lancet*, 372, 1953–61.

Köttgen A, et al. (2013). Genome-wide association analyses identify 18 new loci associated with serum urate concentrations. *Nature Genetics*, 45, 145–54.

Krishnan E, et al. (2012). Nature versus nurture in gout: a twin study. *American Journal of Medicine*, 125, 499–504.

Kuo C-F, et al. (2015). Familial aggregation of gout and relative genetic and environmental contributions: a nationwide population study in Taiwan. *Annals of the Rheumatic Diseases*, 74, 369–74.

Li C, et al. (2015). Genome-wide association analysis identifies three new risk loci for gout arthritis in Han Chinese. *Nature Communications*, 6, art. no. 7041.

Matsuo H, et al. (2015). Genome-wide association study of clinically defined gout identifies multiple risk loci and its association with clinical subtypes. *Annals of the Rheumatic Diseases*. doi: 10.1136/annrheumdis-2014-206191

McAdams-DeMarco MA, et al. (2013). A urate gene-by-diuretic interaction and gout risk in participants with hypertension: results from the ARIC study. *Annals of the Rheumatic Diseases*, 72, 701–6.

Merriman TR, Choi HK, and Dalbeth N (2013). The genetic basis of gout. *Rheumatic Disease Clinics of North America*, 40, 279–90.

Merriman TR (2015). An update on the genetic architecture of hyperuricemia and gout. *Arthritis Research & Therapy*, 17, 98.

Okada Y, et al. (2012). Meta-analysis identifies multiple loci associated with kidney function-related traits in east Asian populations. *Nature Genetics*, 44, 904–9.

Phipps-Green AJ, et al. (2014). Twenty-eight loci that influence serum urate levels: analysis of association with gout. *Annals of the Rheumatic Diseases*. doi: 10.1136/annrheumdis-2014-205877

Qing YF, et al. (2013). Association of TLR4 gene rs2149356 polymorphism with primary gouty arthritis in a case-control study. *PLoS One*, 8, e64845.

Rasheed H, et al. (2013). Association of the lipoprotein receptor-related protein 2 gene with gout and non-additive interaction with alcohol consumption. *Arthritis Research & Therapy*, 15, R177.

Urano W, et al. (2013). Effect of genetic polymorphisms on development of gout. *Journal of Rheumatology*, 40, 1374–78.

Wen CC, et al. (2015). Genome-wide association study identifies ABCG2 (BCRP) as an allopurinol transporter and a determinant of drug response. *Clinical Pharmacology & Therapeutics*, 97, 518–25.

Woodward OM, et al. (2013). Gout-causing Q141K mutation in ABCG2 leads to instability of the nucleotide-binding domain and can be corrected with small molecules. *Proceedings of the National Academy of Sciences of the USA*, 110, 5223–28.

Chapter 5

Clinical features of gout

Key points

- Gout typically presents as recurrent flares of acute self-limiting arthritis.
- The acute gout flare is characterized by severe joint inflammation.
- In the presence of prolonged untreated hyperuricaemia, some people with gout may develop gouty tophi, which cause restricted joint movement, ulceration, and joint damage.
- The differential diagnosis for gout includes septic arthritis (which may co-exist with gout), joint injury, calcium pyrophosphate deposition, basic calcium phosphate arthritis or tendinitis, reactive arthritis, and psoriatic arthritis.

The clinical features of gout are distinctive and have been well described in the medical literature for centuries (Garrod 1859; Hench 1941; Sydenham 1683). More recently, the clinical features of gout have been systematically examined in a large international case-control study using monosodium urate crystal–proven disease as the gold standard (Taylor et al. 2015). This analysis has allowed further quantification of the typical features of gout.

Gout typically presents in middle-aged men. Gout is much less frequent in women and presents in women at an older age, usually after the menopause. Gout is more common in individuals with other features of metabolic syndrome, and in those with chronic kidney disease and cardiovascular disease (see Chapters 3 and 11). A history of kidney stones is present in approximately 10% of people with gout. Blood disorders such as polycythaemia rubra vera are occasionally present. Use of diuretics, particularly loop diuretics, are an important risk factor for development of gout. Other drugs associated with hyperuricaemia and gout include ciclosporin, pyrazinamide, and low-dose aspirin. Up to half of patients describe a family history of gout.

The first presentation of gout is typically an acute inflammatory episode affecting a lower limb joint. Most often the joint is involved, although tendinitis and bursitis can also occur. In approximately half of patients with gout, an acute inflammatory episode in the first metatarsophalangeal joint (podagra) is the first presentation of gout. Other common sites of acute inflammation are the midfoot, ankle, and knee joint.

Acute inflammatory episodes have a stereotypic pattern, with rapid onset of maximal pain within 24 hours of onset and gradual resolution over 1–2 weeks (Bellamy et al. 1987). These episodes often start during the night (Choi et al. 2015). The pain is severe ('the worst pain ever') and associated with joint swelling, warmth, and restricted movement. The joint may be exquisitely tender, and activities such as walking are limited. Joint erythema may also be present at the time of maximal inflammation, and overlying skin may desquamate during the resolution phase. In patients with severe joint inflammation, fever and other systemic symptoms may be present.

In gout, the acute inflammatory episodes are self-limiting. The symptoms and signs of joint inflammation completely disappear, and the patient remains asymptomatic (or back to baseline state) during this 'intercritical period' until the next acute inflammatory episode occurs. A flare of acute inflammation typically occurs a year or so after the first episode. In the absence of treatment, flares occur more frequently over time, involving more joints, including those in the upper limb (including the olecranon bursa). Although spinal disease occasionally complicates advanced gout, the involvement of the spine, hips, and shoulders is uncommon.

Patients may describe triggers of an acute inflammatory episode. These triggers include acute medical or surgical illness, dehydration, and dietary factors such as intake of purine-rich foods or alcohol. Acute inflammatory episodes are also more common at times of high ambient temperature and extremes of humidity (Neogi et al. 2014). Joint injury or overuse is another frequent trigger, with onset of acute inflammation some hours after the joint injury.

In the presence of persistent hyperuricaemia, chronic gouty arthritis may develop over time. Chronic gouty arthritis manifests as nonresolving synovitis, gouty tophi, and joint damage. In the absence of urate-lowering therapy, this presentation typically occurs approximately ten years after presentation of the first acute inflammatory episode, although there is wide variation in this interval: some patients present with chronic gouty arthritis as the first manifestation of disease; others never develop tophi despite persistently high serum urate concentrations and recurrent acute inflammatory episodes. Patients with chronic kidney disease are more likely to develop tophi early in disease.

Tophi have been defined as 'draining or chalk-like subcutaneous nodules under transparent skin, often with overlying vascularity, located in typical locations: joints, ears, olecranon bursae, finger pads, tendons (e.g. Achilles)' (Neogi et al. 2015) (see Figures 5.1 and 5.2). Tophi are usually nontender, but may become acutely inflamed with associated tenderness. These lesions may cause joint deformity and obstruction to joint movement. Foot tophi may lead to difficulty finding shoes. The presence of hand tophi is strongly associated with impaired grip strength

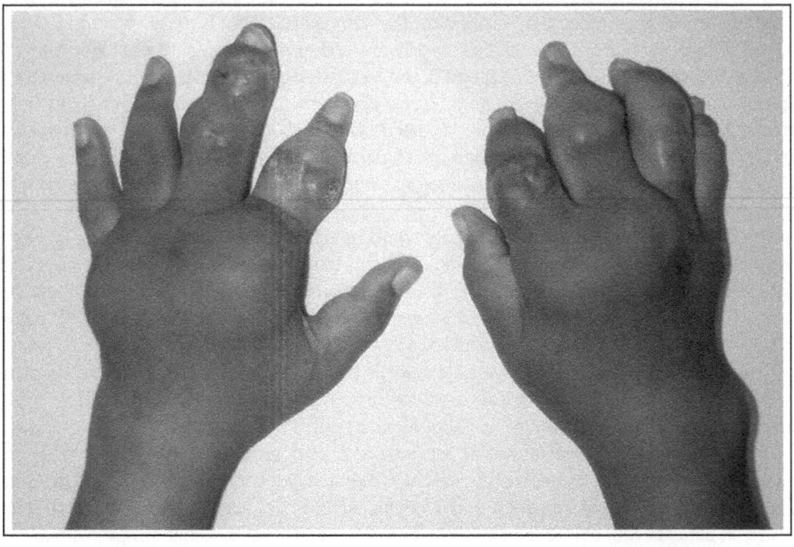

Figure 5.1 Severe tophaceous gout affecting the hands. Note the numerous discharging tophi. Adapted with permission from Dalbeth et al. *Arthritis & Rheumatism* 2007.

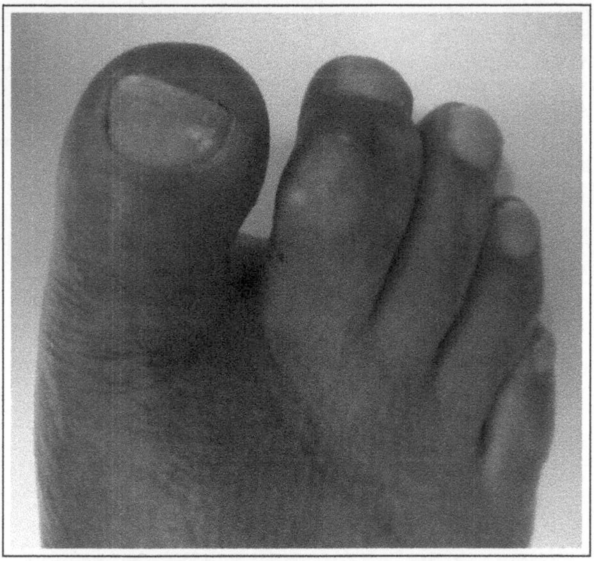

Figure 5.2 Tophus affecting the right second toe.
Adapted with permission from Dalbeth et al. *Annals of the Rheumatic Diseases* 2011.

and difficulty with functional grips. Intraosseous tophi lead to bone erosion. Discharging tophi may develop superimposed infection.

The differential diagnosis of an acute inflammatory episode due to gout includes other causes of acute monoarthritis. The most important is septic arthritis (which may co-exist with gout). Other important differential diagnoses are joint trauma, calcium pyrophosphate deposition, basic calcium phosphate arthritis or tendinitis, reactive arthritis, and psoriatic arthritis. Although osteoarthritis may also affect the first metatarsophalangeal joint, it is usually not difficult to differentiate gout and osteoarthritis, based on the degree of joint inflammation and temporal course of disease. Similarly, gout can usually be distinguished from rheumatoid arthritis, due to the history of intermittent acute inflammatory episodes and pattern of joint involvement. Gouty tophi can be distinguished from other subcutaneous nodules or swellings, such as rheumatoid nodules, lipid deposits, and osteophytes, due to the typical appearance and characteristic locations. Laboratory tests including serum urate testing and particularly joint or nodule aspiration play a key role in differentiating between gout and other rheumatic diseases, as described in Chapter 6.

References

Bellamy N, Downie WW, Buchanan WW (1987). Observations on spontaneous improvement in patients with podagra: implications for therapeutic trials of non-steroidal anti-inflammatory drugs. *British Journal of Clinical Pharmacology*, 24(1), 33–6.

Choi HK, et al. (2015). Nocturnal risk of gout attacks. *Arthritis & Rheumatatology*, 67(2), 555–62.

Garrod AB (1859). *The nature and treatment of gout and rheumatic gout*. Walton and Maberly, London.

Hench PS (1941). Diagnosis and treatment of gout and gouty arthritis. *Journal of the American Medical Association*, 116(6), 453–59.

Neogi T, et al. (2014). Relation of temperature and humidity to the risk of recurrent gout attacks. *American Journal of Epidemiology*, 180(4), 372–7.

Neogi T, et al. (2015). 2015 gout classification criteria: an American College of Rheumatology/European League Against Rheumatism collaborative initiative. *Arthritis & Rheumatology*, 67(10), 2557–2568.

Sydenham T (1683). *A treatise of the gout and dropsy*. G. Kettilby, London.

Taylor WJ, et al. (2015). Study for Updated Gout Classification Criteria (SUGAR): identification of features to classify gout. *Arthritis Care & Research (Hoboken)*, 67(9), 1304–15.

Chapter 6

Laboratory testing in gout diagnosis and management

Key points

- Identification of monosodium urate (MSU) crystals is the gold standard for gout diagnosis.
- Serum urate is an important test for both gout diagnosis and effective management.
- For people with gout on urate-lowering therapy, the target urate concentration is less than 0.36 mmol/L (6 mg/dL).
- Blood tests may also assist with screening for co-morbid conditions in gout.
- Urine tests may assist in determining the basis for hyperuricaemia in people with gout.
- Microscopically, the tophus represents a chronic inflammatory granulomatous response to MSU crystal aggregates.

Laboratory tests are important both for accurate diagnosis and effective and safe management of gout. Most important are serum urate testing and microscopic examination for MSU crystal identification. Urine testing is also useful to understand the underlying basis of hyperuricaemia in people with gout. Other blood tests may assist with screening of co-morbid conditions and monitoring for drug safety.

6.1 Blood testing

6.1.1 Serum urate

Serum urate is tested on venous blood in a chemical pathology laboratory, using a uricase assay, a method with high reliability and precision (Miller et al. 2008). No clinically important diurnal variation exists for serum urate, and it can be measured non-fasting at any time of day.

For gout diagnosis, an elevated serum urate level in an individual with arthritis increases the likelihood of gout, but is not diagnostic. The presence of a serum urate concentration consistently below 0.36 mmol/L (6 mg/dL) substantially reduces the likelihood of gout; in a recent large multinational study of people presenting with at least one swollen joint or subcutaneous nodule, only 7% of those with crystal-proven gout had serum urate levels consistently below 0.36 mmol/L (Taylor et al. 2015). Up to 40% of patients with an acute gout flare may have serum urate within the normal range (Logan et al. 1997). Therefore, if the serum urate is not elevated at the time of a flare of arthritis and the diagnosis of gout remains a possibility, testing should be repeated after the acute inflammatory episode has resolved to help establish the diagnosis of gout.

Serum urate testing is essential for monitoring of gout treatment. For all people with gout on urate-lowering therapy, the target concentration is less than 0.36 mmol/L (6 mg/dL). This target is recommended by both the American College of Rheumatology (ACR) and the European League Against Rheumatism (EULAR) (Khanna et al. 2012; Zhang et al. 2006), and is required to achieve MSU crystal dissolution in vivo, prevent acute inflammatory episodes, and allow regression of tophi. The velocity of tophus regression is inversely related to the serum urate concentration (Perez-Ruiz et al. 2002); for this reason, a lower target—less than 0.30 mmol/L (5 mg/dL)—may be required for those with severe tophaceous disease. Monitoring of serum urate concentration is crucial to ensure that patients are achieving the relevant treatment target and to guide intensification of urate-lowering therapy to achieve the target.

6.1.2 **Other blood tests**

Inflammatory markers such as the C-reactive protein are typically elevated during the acute inflammatory episode in gout (Roseff et al. 1987). The C-reactive protein is often elevated >100 mg/L, and is typically higher if large joints are affected or in the case of a polyarthritis. This test is non-specific and reflects the degree of joint inflammation rather than gout itself. The C-reactive protein may be similarly elevated in any other form of arthritis, including septic arthritis and other forms of crystal arthritis. The C-reactive protein is typically normal between acute inflammatory episodes during the intercritical period, and may be mildly elevated in patients with chronic tophaceous gouty arthropathy.

At the time of diagnosis, and periodically during treatment of people with gout, screening for co-morbid conditions is indicated (Zhang et al. 2006). Blood testing for co-morbid conditions includes serum creatinine (for chronic kidney disease), HbA1c or fasting glucose (for type 2 diabetes), and lipid profile (for cardiovascular risk assessment).

*HLA-B*5801* is strongly associated with severe cutaneous adverse reactions due to allopurinol, and *HLA-B*5801* testing has been advocated for screening in populations with high allele frequency (e.g. Han Chinese, Korean, Thai) prior to commencement of allopurinol (Khanna et al. 2012). If positive, avoidance of allopurinol and selection of an alternative urate-lowering drug is recommended. For those on drug therapies for gout management, blood tests may also be required for safety monitoring. For those on long-term colchicine prophylaxis, full blood count and CK monitoring may be required, particularly in people with kidney disease (Mikuls et al. 2004). For those on febuxostat or benzbromarone, periodic liver function test monitoring is required.

6.2 **Assessment of renal excretion (fractional excretion of urate and urinary urate excretion)**

Various methods of assessing renal excretion have been described (Simkin 2001). Although assessment of 24-hour urinary uric acid excretion (UUE) has traditionally been considered the gold standard for assessment of renal excretion, there can be marked intra-individual variation between samples. UUE can be normalized for a body surface area of 1.73 m^2. Ideally, this test should be obtained following a low-purine, low-fructose, low-alcohol, and calorie-controlled diet.

An alternative approach for screening for over-excretion is the Simkin index, which allows analysis of a spot urine specimen. It is recommended that this sample is obtained midmorning after a light, low-purine, low-fructose breakfast, and without a preceding exercise session.

The Simkin index is calculated as the product of the urinary uric acid concentration and the plasma creatinine divided by the urinary creatinine, which yields the excretion rate per unit of glomerular filtrate $([U_{urate} \times P_{creatinine}] \div U_{creatinine})$. The normal adult mean is 0.4 (± 0.1 SD) mg of urinary uric acid per decilitre of glomerular filtrate. If the value is greater than 0.6 mg/dL, it is recommended that the test be repeated. If a high level is found again, then a 24-hour testing is recommended.

Another widely used measurement of urinary uric acid handling is the fractional excretion of urate (FEUA), which represents the urate clearance/creatinine clearance ratio $([U_{urate} \times P_{creatinine}] \div [U_{creatinine} \times P_{urate}])$.

The causes of hyperuricaemia have been classified into three groups based on these results: (a) overproduction hyperuricaemia, with UUE >25.0 mg $h^{-1}/1.73\ m^2$ (600 mg per day/1.73 m^2) and FEUA ≥5.5%; (b) under-excretion hyperuricaemia, with UUE ≤25.0 mg $h^{-1}/1.73\ m^2$ and FEUA <5.5%; and (c) a combined type with UUE>25.0 mg $h^{-1}/1.73\ m^2$ and FEUA<5.5%. It has been suggested recently that analysis of *ABCG2* genotypes may allow further separation of urate overproduction/combined types into genuine overproduction and extra-renal under-excretion (Ichida et al. 2012).

6.3 Synovial fluid analysis

Synovial fluid analysis in suspected gout includes assessment of macroscopic synovial fluid appearance; cell count; differential, microbiological analysis (Gram stain and culture); and microscopy for crystal identification. (Pascual and Jovani 2005).

In acute gouty arthritis, synovial fluid is typically non-viscous, yellow, and cloudy. The white cell count is in the inflammatory range and may be greater than 50,000 cells/mm^3, predominantly (>90%) neutrophils. In uninflamed intercritical joints, synovial fluid is viscous, clear, and yellow with cell count <2000 cells/mm^3, with a lower proportion of neutrophils.

Gout and septic arthritis can co-exist. Therefore, even in a person with an established diagnosis of gout, aspirated synovial fluid obtained from an acutely inflamed joint should be assessed routinely for microbiological testing.

Synovial fluid crystals that are routinely detected in clinical practice are MSU and calcium pyrophosphate (CPP). Although MSU crystals can be detected 48 hours after sample collection, analysis of fresh synovial fluid samples is recommended, particularly for CPP crystal identification. A small drop of fluid is placed on a glass slide and covered with a cover slip. For compensated light microscopy, the microscope is fitted with two polarizing filters, one below (polarizer) and one above (analyzer) the stage, and a first-order red compensator. Using this system, MSU crystals are visualized as needle-shaped, negatively birefringent crystals (yellow when parallel to the compensator axis and blue when perpendicular to it; see Figure 6.1). In synovial fluid, MSU crystals range in size between 1–20 μm. MSU crystals may be intracellular, extracellular, or both. In contrast, CPP crystals are visualized as weakly positive rhomboid-shaped crystals; these crystals may be quite faint and needle-shaped on occasion. MSU and CPP crystals may co-exist.

Although crystal identification is most often undertaken in accredited microbiology laboratories, examination of synovial fluid for crystal identification is still practised in some rheumatology clinics. If MSU crystals are identified, this testing allows rapid diagnosis of gout. Testing has the further advantage of allowing patients with gout to visualize MSU crystals, which can be an important tool for patient understanding of the importance of long-term urate-lowering therapy to achieve dissolution of crystals. Appropriate training is required in order to achieve

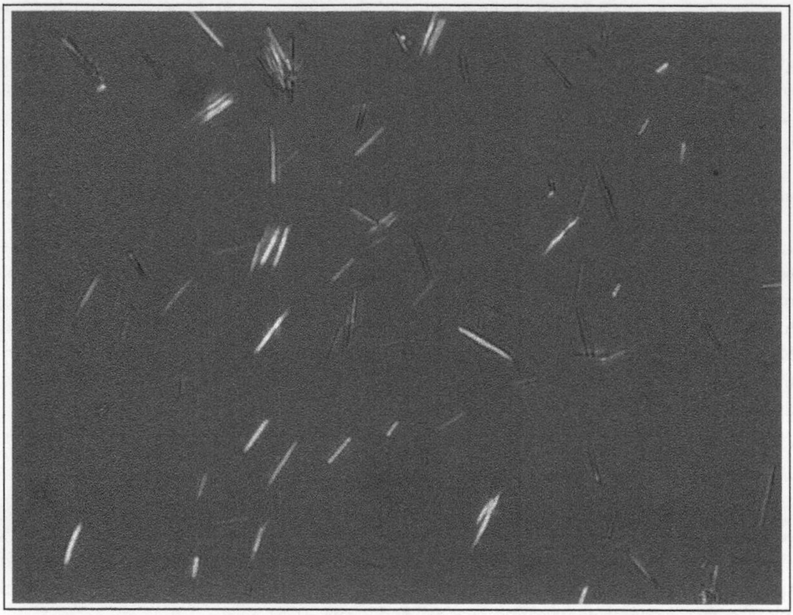

Figure 6.1 Aspirated MSU crystals observed under polarizing light microscopy, magnification ×40. Note the needle-shaped negatively birefringent crystals. (See colour version on inside cover.)

and maintain competency in crystal identification; both EULAR and ACR offer crystal identification workshops to facilitate this training.

6.4 Tophus analysis: microscopy and histology

MSU crystals can also be identified following needle aspiration from a tophus or by swabbing a discharging tophus. Using polarizing light microscopy, MSU crystals can frequently be identified in tophus samples processed for histology. When a resected nodule is suspicious for a tophus, the pathological sample should ideally be processed in ethanol rather than formalin to avoid dissolution of MSU crystals during processing. MSU crystals are typically larger within tophi (up to 40 μm in length) and are densely packed into bundles (Figure 6.2).

Histologically, the tophus represents a chronic inflammatory granulomatous response, with islands of MSU crystal aggregates each surrounded by a cellular rim or 'corona zone' consisting of macrophages, multinucleated giant cells, mast cells, and plasma cells (Figure 6.3) (Dalbeth et al. 2010; Sokoloff 1957). Cytokines such as IL-1 and TNFα are expressed within the corona zone. A fibrovascular zone surrounds the corona zone, consisting of blood vessels and dense connective tissue. Cells within the fibrovascular zone include scattered macrophages, T cells, B cells, mast cells, and plasma cells.

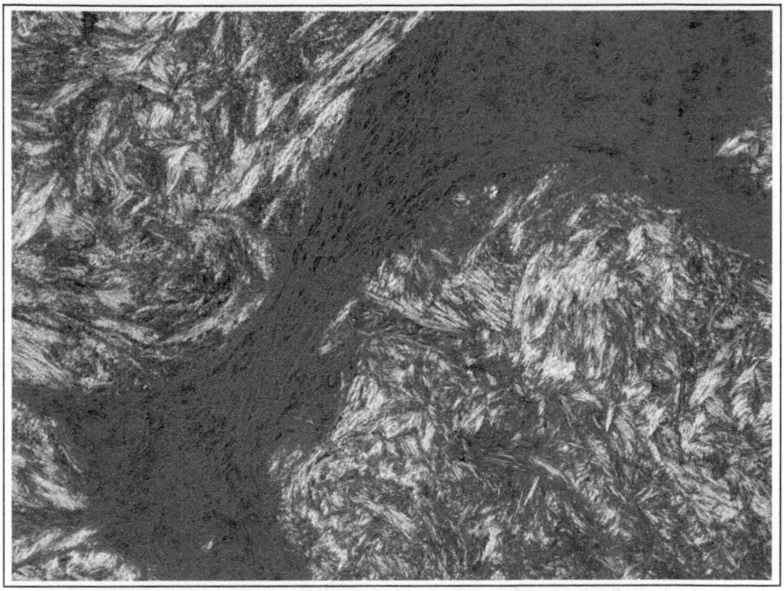

Figure 6.2 Formalin-fixed tophus sample under polarizing light microscopy, prior to processing for histology, demonstrating islands of tightly packed MSU crystals, magnification ×20. (See colour version on inside cover.)

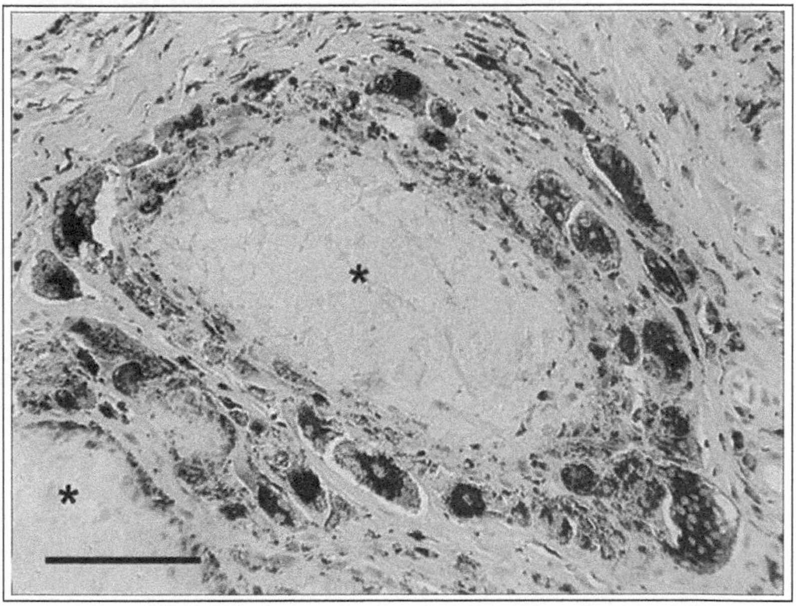

Figure 6.3 Immunohistochemistry of the tophus for CD68. Positively staining mononucleated and multinucleated cells are observed in the cellular corona zone surrounding the MSU crystal core (denoted as *), magnification ×20. (See colour version on inside cover.)

Adapted with permission from Dalbeth N, et al. (2010). Cellular characterization of the gouty tophus: a quantitative analysis. *Arthritis & Rheumatism*, 62(5), 1549–56.

References

Dalbeth N, et al. (2010). Cellular characterization of the gouty tophus: a quantitative analysis. *Arthritis & Rheumatism*, 62(5), 1549–56.

Ichida K, et al. (2012). Decreased extra-renal urate excretion is a common cause of hyperuricemia. *Nature Communications*, 3, art. no. 764.

Khanna D, et al. (2012). 2012 American College of Rheumatology guidelines for management of gout. Part 1: systematic nonpharmacologic and pharmacologic therapeutic approaches to hyperuricemia. *Arthritis Care & Research (Hoboken)*, 64(10), 1431–46.

Logan JA, Morrison E, McGill PE (1997). Serum uric acid in acute gout. *Annals of the Rheumatic Diseases*, 56(11), 696–7.

Mikuls TR, et al. (2004). Quality of care indicators for gout management. *Arthritis & Rheumatism*, 50(3), 937–43.

Miller WG, et al. (2008). State of the art in trueness and interlaboratory harmonization for 10 analytes in general clinical chemistry. *Archives of Pathology & Laboratory Medicine*, 132(5), 838–46.

Pascual E and Jovani V (2005). Synovial fluid analysis. *Best Practice & Research: Clinical Rheumatology*, 19(3), 371–86.

Perez-Ruiz F, et al. (2002). Effect of urate-lowering therapy on the velocity of size reduction of tophi in chronic gout. *Arthritis & Rheumatism*, 47(4), 356–60.

Roseff R, et al. (1987). The acute phase response in gout. *Journal of Rheumatology*, 14(5), 974–7.

Simkin PA (2001). When, why, and how should we quantify the excretion rate of urinary uric acid? *Journal of Rheumatology*, 28(6), 1207–10.

Sokoloff L (1957). The pathology of gout. *Metabolism*, 6(3), 230–43.

Taylor WJ, et al. (2015). Study for Updated Gout Classification Criteria (SUGAR): identification of features to classify gout. *Arthritis Care & Research (Hoboken)*, 67(9), 1304–15.

Zhang W, et al. (2006). EULAR evidence based recommendations for gout. Part II: Management. Report of a task force of the EULAR Standing Committee for International Clinical Studies Including Therapeutic (ESCISIT). *Annals of the Rheumatic Diseases*, 65(10), 1312–24.

Chapter 7

Imaging in gout

Key points

- Plain radiographic changes of gout such as erosion and joint space narrowing occur late in the course of disease.
- Advanced imaging methods have provided new insights into the pathology of gout.
- Ultrasonography is able to detect features of urate crystal deposition, including the double contour sign and tophus.
- Dual energy CT also allows detection and quantification of urate deposits.
- CT and MRI have clinical utility in assessing for disease complications in gout.

In addition to laboratory testing (Chapter 6), radiological tests may assist in diagnosis and monitoring of gout. There are five main imaging modalities routinely used in clinical practice: plain radiography, ultrasonography (US), magnetic resonance imaging (MRI), conventional computed tomography (CT), and dual energy CT (DECT). The key findings that can be detected by each of these modalities in people with gout are shown in Table 7.1. These modalities differ from each other in availability, cost, requirement for ionizing radiation, and the ability to detect pathological features of gout. This chapter will review each imaging modality in the context of gout diagnosis and monitoring.

7.1 Plain radiography

Plain radiography is the most widely available imaging modality in clinical practice. Soft tissue swelling (due to synovitis or tophus), bone erosion, new bone formation (spurs, sclerosis, periosteal new bone formation) and joint space abnormalities (narrowing, widening, and occasionally ankylosis) can be detected by plain radiography (Figure 7.1) (Bloch et al. 1980; Dalbeth et al. 2012a). Plain radiographic bone erosion in gout has a typical appearance that has been defined as 'a cortical break with sclerotic margin and overhanging edge' (Neogi et al. 2015). In contrast to other forms of erosive arthritis, bone density adjacent to the erosion is well maintained, and bone sclerosis at the edge of the erosion is usually observed. A further distinctive feature of radiographic damage in gout is that joint space narrowing is typically a late feature. Bone erosion preferentially occurs at characteristic sites in gout, particularly in the feet affecting the first metatarsophalangeal joint (MTPJ), fifth MTPJ, and midfoot (mirroring the sites of acute gouty inflammation that present clinically). In advanced disease, erosions may be present at many other joints, including the hands and wrists. Involvement of soft tissues is not well defined by plain radiography, although the consequences of ligament disruption may be observed—for example, scapholunate dissociation at the wrist.

Table 7.1 Pathological features in gout detected by various imaging modalities

Imaging modality	Pathological feature	Typical appearance
Radiography	Tophus	Soft tissue mass
	Erosion	Well-demarcated, corticated, over-hanging margin, intra-articular and extra-articular sites
	Joint space abnormalities	Include narrowing, widening, ankylosis
	New bone formation	Spur, sclerosis, periosteal new bone formation
Ultrasonography	MSU crystal deposition	The double contour sign defined as 'hyperechoic irregular enhancement over the surface of the hyaline cartilage that is independent of the insonation angle of the ultrasound beam'
	Joint effusion	May have 'snowstorm' appearance due to MSU crystals within synovial fluid
	Tophus	Hyperechoic, heterogeneous lesion surrounded by an anechoic rim
	Aggregates	Hyperechoic dots present within synovium, tendon, and other joint structures
	Synovitis	Synovial hypertrophy with power Doppler flow
	Tendon pathology	Includes tenosynovitis, tendinosis, enthesitis, and intratendinous tophus
	Erosion	Cortical break present in two planes
MRI	Joint effusion	Low signal on T1w images, homogenous high signal on T2w images, no contrast enhancement
	Synovitis	An area in the synovial compartment that shows enhancement with contrast with a thickness greater than the width of the normal synovium
	Tendon pathology	Includes tenosynovitis, tendinosis, and intratendinous tophus
	Tophus	Mass with intermediate signal intensity appearance on T1w images, but more variability on T2w images. Variable contrast enhancement at tophus border. Contrast not required to assess tophus volume
	Erosion	A sharply marginated bone lesion with loss of normal low-signal intensity of cortical bone and loss of normal high-signal intensity of trabecular bone on non-fat-suppressed T1w images

(*continued*)

Table 7.1 Continued

Imaging modality	Pathological feature	Typical appearance
	Bone marrow oedema	Lesion within trabecular bone with ill-defined margins and demonstrating low signal intensity on T1w images, increased signal intensity on T2w images, and enhancement with contrast Typically adjacent to tophus in uncomplicated gout
	Cartilage pathology	Includes focal and diffuse narrowing
Conventional CT	Tophus	Soft tissue mass, typically 170 Hounsfield units
	Erosion	Well-demarcated, corticated, overhanging margin, intra-articular and extra-articular sites
	New bone formation	Spur, sclerosis, periosteal new bone formation
DECT	MSU crystal deposition	Urate differentially colour coded, plus conventional CT features

Source: Modified from Dalbeth COR 2011.

Plain radiographic changes are not typically present at the time of first presentation of gout; they usually develop years after onset of disease in those who have had untreated hyperuricaemia. The presence of subcutaneous tophi is strongly associated with the presence of bone erosion, new bone formation, and joint space narrowing in people with gout. Typically, gout diagnosis is not a challenge in those with long-standing disease with clinically apparent tophi, and in this context, plain radiography is not usually required to establish a diagnosis of gout. However, in occasional atypical presentations of chronic gouty arthritis, the presence of typical radiographic changes may provide useful diagnostic information.

The 2012 American College of Rheumatology Gout Management Guidelines advise that presence of typical radiographic damage is a clear indication for urate-lowering therapy. Therefore, assessing plain radiographs may be useful when considering whether a patient should be commenced on urate-lowering therapy.

A quantitative scoring system has been established for monitoring of structural damage in gout, which is a modification of the Sharp–van der Heijde method for rheumatoid arthritis scoring (Dalbeth et al. 2007a). This method is reproducible, and has high face and construct validity. Scores are typically higher in patients with subcutaneous tophi and in those with longer disease duration. Bone and joint damage scored using this method correlates highly with measures of musculoskeletal disability. To date, structure modification using plain radiography has not been reported in clinical trials of gout. In a small longitudinal study of pegloticase in people with advanced gout, very intensive urate-lowering therapy was associated with regression of bone erosion (Dalbeth et al. 2014). At present it is not clear what serum urate target is required to achieve this outcome, or whether it can be achieved with available oral urate-lowering therapies.

7.2 Ultrasonography

Ultrasonography (US) is widely adopted within rheumatology practice, and does not require ionizing radiation. In addition to the standard features that can be identified on

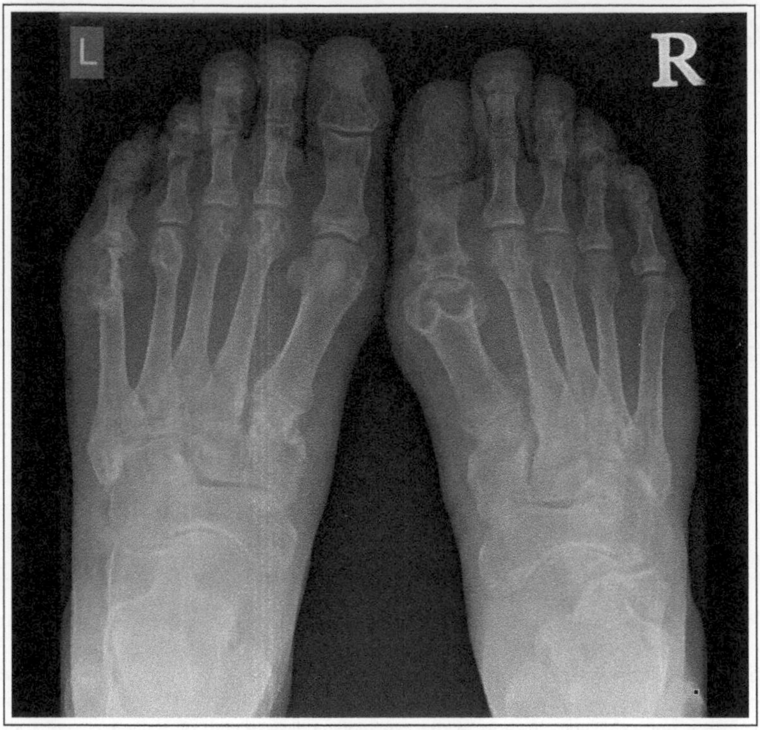

Figure 7.1 Plain radiographs of the feet in a patient with tophaceous gout, demonstrating typical gouty erosions. Note the associated soft tissue density, sclerotic margin, and overhanging edge. These images show the classical distribution of gouty erosions, affecting the first and fifth metatarsophalangeal joints, and midfoot joints.

Adapted with permission from Dalbeth, N., et al. *Ann Rheum Dis*. 2015 Jun;74(6):1030–6.

musculoskeletal US in other inflammatory arthropathies, such as synovial hypertrophy, power Doppler signal, erosions, and tendon and enthesial pathology, features specific to gout have also been identified (Grassi et al. 2006; Thiele and Schlesinger 2007) (Figures 7.2 and 7.3). These features are thought to represent monosodium urate (MSU) crystals in different states within the joint, including the double contour sign (defined as hyperechoic irregular enhancement over the surface of the hyaline cartilage that is independent of the insonation angle of the ultrasound beam [Neogi et al. 2015] representing MSU crystals overlying the articular cartilage); small aggregates of urate (which may represent 'microtophi'); snowstorm appearance (representing MSU crystals within the synovial fluid); and the tophus (an organized structure which includes both MSU crystal aggregates and the chronic inflammatory response to these crystals).

US may have particular utility for gout diagnosis. Its first role is to guide aspiration of synovial fluid for the gold standard of gout diagnosis: microscopic identification of MSU crystals. US may assist with identification of joint effusions and selection of sites for aspiration. In addition, some US features are considered highly specific for gout, and may allow a diagnosis of gout in the absence of microscopically proven disease. In a multicentre study of US in 824 people

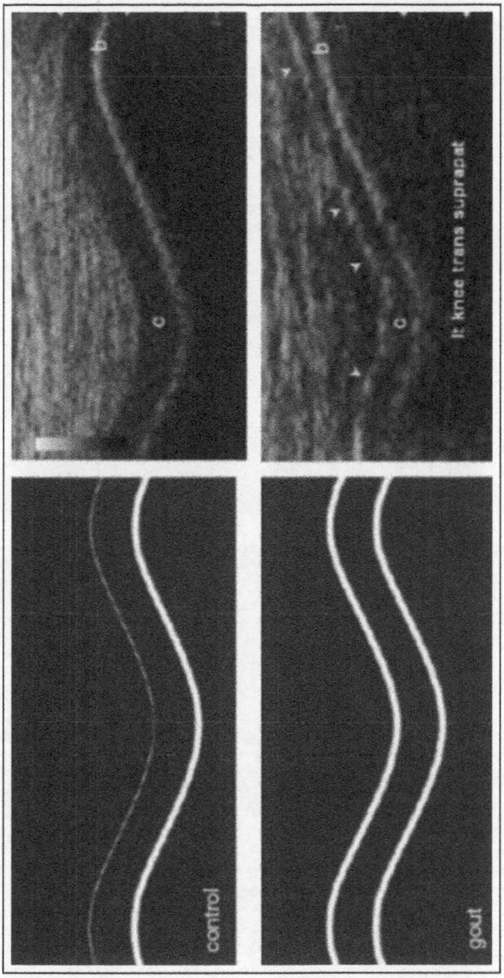

Figure 7.2 The ultrasound double contour sign in gout. Ultrasound appearances of articular cartilage in the knee in a normal subject and in gout, according to the model described by Thiele and Schlesinger (2007). MSU crystals overlie the surface of articular cartilage, leading to the double contour sign in gout. Arrows indicate irregular MSU crystal deposits over the surface of articular cartilage. c: cartilage, b: bone.

Adapted with permission from Thiele, R. G. and Schlesinger, N. (2007), Diagnosis of gout by ultrasound, Rheumatology (Oxford), 46 (7), 1116–21.

presenting with joint swelling, which involved scanning of the affected joint, high specificity for gout was observed for double contour sign and US tophus, when compared to MSU crystal identification as the gold standard (Ogdie et al. 2015). In those with early disease (defined as onset of first episode within two years), the specificity for double contour sign was 92.3%, but the sensitivity was only 50.9%. Similar high specificity was observed in this group for US tophus (95.4%) and snowstorm appearance (92.3%), with even lower sensitivity (33.6% for US

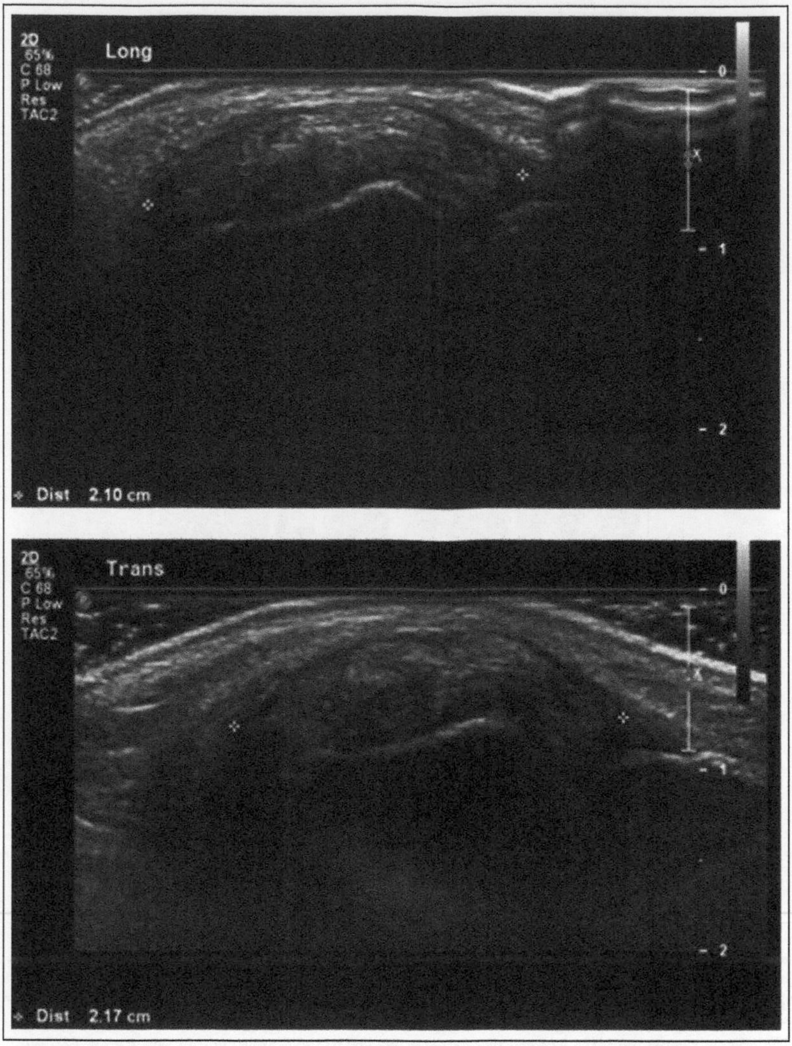

Figure 7.3 The ultrasound tophus in gout. Ultrasound image of the first metatarsophalangeal joint. Measurement of longest tophus diameters measured in the longitudinal (upper panel) and transverse (lower panel) axes.

Adapted with permission from Dalbeth et al. (2011), *Annals of the Rheumatic Diseases.*

tophus and 32.4% for snowstorm appearance). For all of these features, sensitivity was lower in those without clinically apparent tophaceous disease (for double contour sign 53.4%, for US tophus 29.4%, and for snowstorm appearance 24.1%), confirming that those with clinically apparent evidence of MSU crystal deposition are more likely to have US evidence of MSU crystal deposition. Despite these limitations, the high specificity indicates that, when present, a positive US feature can provide valuable supportive evidence of gout, including in those with recent onset of disease.

It is important to note that, although more frequent in those with symptomatic disease, some features of MSU crystal deposition on US (double contour sign and tophus) are also present in those with asymptomatic hyperuricaemia who have never experienced an acute arthritis. Overall, these features are present in approximately 25% of people with serum urate concentrations of 0.48 mmol/L or higher (Pineda et al. 2011). It is currently unknown whether asymptomatic individuals with hyperuricaemia and US features of MSU crystal deposition are at higher risk of developing symptomatic disease than hyperuricaemic individuals who do not have these US features. Furthermore, there are no data supporting the treatment of asymptomatic individuals with hyperuricaemia and US features of MSU crystal deposition.

In patients with established gout, US may assist with identification of MSU crystal deposition at sites that are not readily clinically visible, including tendons and ligaments (Naredo et al. 2014). In addition to features of MSU crystal deposition, US may demonstrate features of subclinical inflammation in both synovium and tendon in people with gout. Bone erosion that is not apparent on plain radiography may also be evident on US.

US may play a role in monitoring clinical response to urate-lowering therapy. A few small studies have reported that the double contour sign can resolve after months of effective urate-lowering therapy. US tophus responds to urate-lowering therapy: a study of people with gout commencing urate-lowering therapy reported a strong linear inverse relationship between change in US tophus maximum diameter and volume and average serum urate concentrations over a 12-month period (Perez-Ruiz et al. 2007).

7.3 Magnetic resonance imaging (MRI)

Although MRI is used in clinical practice, this modality is used less frequently than plain radiography and US due to cost and time required for scanning. Positioning for adequate views can also be difficult in those with joint pain or structural damage. The use of contrast can also be problematic in people with gout, who frequently have co-morbid chronic kidney disease.

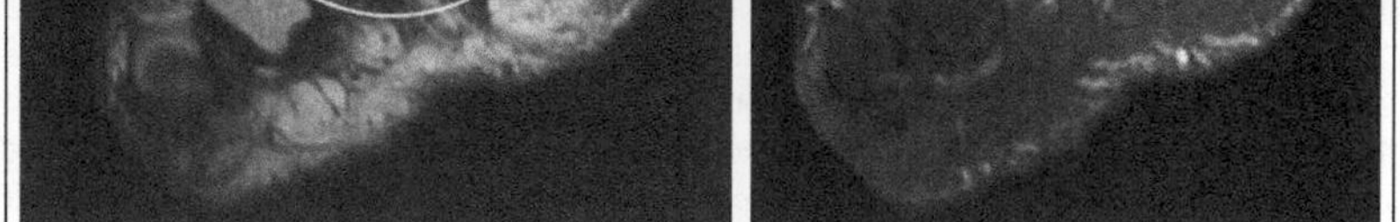

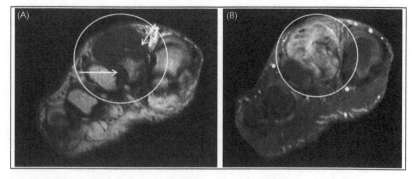

Figure 7.4 MRI scan of the gouty tophus. A: pre-contrast; B: post-contrast. Axial T1w MRI scans of the forefoot show a large tophus (circle) involving the head of the second metatarsal. The tophus enhances with contrast and there are associated erosions (arrows) directly adjacent.

Adapted with permission from Poh, Y. J., et al. (2011), Magnetic resonance imaging bone edema is not a major feature of gout unless there is concomitant osteomyelitis: 10-year findings from a high-prevalence population, J Rheumatol, 38 (11), 2475–81.

On MRI, the tophus is visualized as a mass with intermediate signal intensity appearance on T1w images, but more variability on T2w images (Yu et al. 1997) (Figure 7.4). Following contrast, there is variable enhancement at tophus border. Tophi may be visualized at intra-articular and extra-articular sites on MRI, including excellent visualization of tendon involvement. On MRI, tophi are visualized along compartmental and fascial lines, but, when large, may penetrate through focal discontinuities of superficial fascial layers or deeper compartmental fascial planes (Popp et al. 1996). MRI tophus volume can be measured using manual outlining techniques. This method does not require contrast, has high concurrent validity with US tophus size, is able to assess both intra-articular and subcutaneous tophi, and has excellent inter-reader reproducibility.

The diagnostic accuracy of MRI for gout has not been reported to date. Although tophi can be identified, MRI is not able to specifically detect MSU crystals. A small study has compared MRI findings in eight patients with acute gout flares affecting the wrist with eight patients with active rheumatoid arthritis (RA) (Cimmino et al. 2011). All patients with acute gout and RA had synovitis, bone marrow oedema, and bone erosions (sensitivity for gout 1.0, specificity 0.0). These data suggest that the MRI findings in acute gout flares may not be sufficiently specific to differentiate between other forms of inflammatory arthritis.

MRI demonstrates high prevalence of synovitis in people with gout, particularly during an acute gout flare (Cimmino et al. 2011), but also in very early disease and in those without clinically inflamed joints. MRI synovitis is responsive to urate-lowering therapy, suggesting that MSU crystals within the joint induce low-grade, chronic synovitis (Dalbeth et al. 2015). MRI also allows excellent detection of bone erosions, which are strongly associated with tophi but not with synovitis or bone marrow oedema (McQueen et al. 2014). Bone marrow oedema may be present during acute gouty arthritis, but is infrequently observed in patients without acute flares, even when subclinical synovitis and erosion is present.

Cartilage damage in gout can also be observed using MRI; compared with RA, this damage is typically mild and focal. Cartilage damage in gout is closely related to tophi, synovitis, and erosion, but not to bone marrow oedema (Popovich et al. 2014).

As with other advanced imaging modalities, MRI is often used for assessment of complications of disease in patients with established gout (Poh et al. 2011). In addition to assessment of joint damage, these include investigation of spinal involvement; assessment of soft tissue disease, such as carpal tunnel syndrome and tendon rupture; and investigation of large soft tissue masses. MRI may also have particular utility in the context of a severe acute inflammatory arthritis presentation when exclusion of soft tissue or bone infection is required. The presence of florid bone marrow oedema in this situation is strongly suggestive of osteomyelitis and necessitates careful exclusion of infection.

7.4 Conventional CT

Conventional CT is not widely used in clinical practice for assessment of gout, due to the requirement for ionizing radiation, unlike other advanced imaging methods such as US and MRI. However, this method does provide excellent visualization of tophi and is considered the gold standard for assessment of bone disease. On CT, the tophus is typically visualized as a soft tissue mass, with a density of 170 HU (Figure 7.5) (Gerster et al. 1996). Although assessment of tophus size using standard CT software has excellent reproducibility and validity, physical measurement of index subcutaneous tophi using Vernier calipers has similar reproducibility and correlates highly with CT measurement, suggesting that simpler methods may be sufficient for monitoring of tophaceous disease (Dalbeth et al. 2007b).

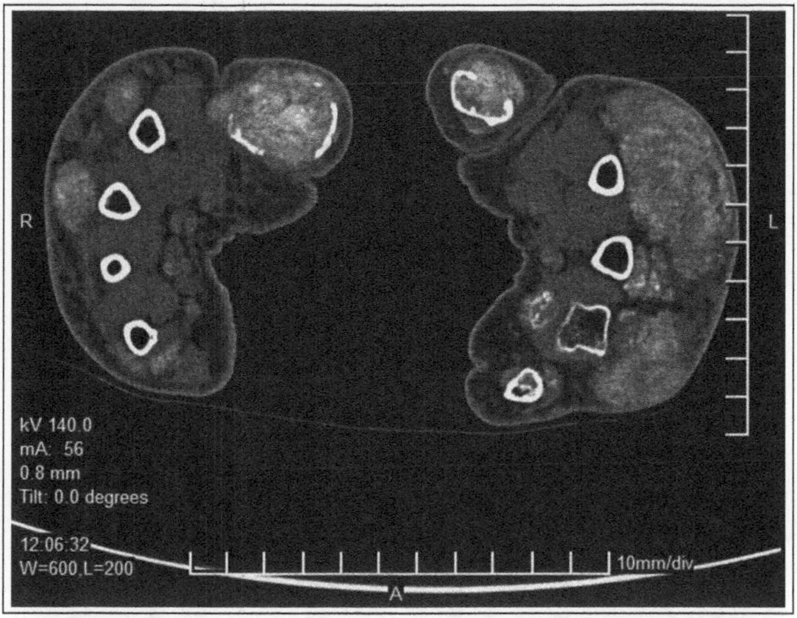

Figure 7.5 Conventional CT of the hands in a patient with severe tophaceous gout. Axial 2D CT images show intraosseous tophi associated with bone erosion.

CT provides excellent visualization of bone erosion and also features of new bone formation, including spur formation, sclerosis, and periosteal new bone formation (Dalbeth et al. 2012a). CT bone erosion scores are strongly associated with the presence of tophaceous disease and other measures of severe gout. The close relationship between intraosseous tophus and bone erosion in individual bones has also been demonstrated using conventional CT (Dalbeth et al. 2009).

Conventional CT has been reported as a useful tool for assessment of spinal disease, due to its ability to visualize both tophus and erosion. A study of 48 patients with poorly controlled gout reported that over one-third had axial erosion and/or tophi on CT scanning of the cervical and lumbosacral spine (Konatalapalli et al. 2012). Disease was observed most frequently in the lumbar spine. There was no clear relationship between the presence of axial involvement on CT and symptoms of back pain.

7.5 Dual energy CT

Dual energy CT (DECT) determines the composition of different tissues by analyzing the difference in attenuation in a material exposed to two different X-ray spectra (typically 80 and 140 kVp) simultaneously (Nicolaou et al. 2010). This method uses algorithms that assign different colours to materials of different chemical composition.

The ability to differentially colour code urate and calcium was originally validated as a non-invasive method to determine the chemical composition of kidney stones (Graser et al. 2008). More recently, this method has been used to identify urate for diagnosis and assessment

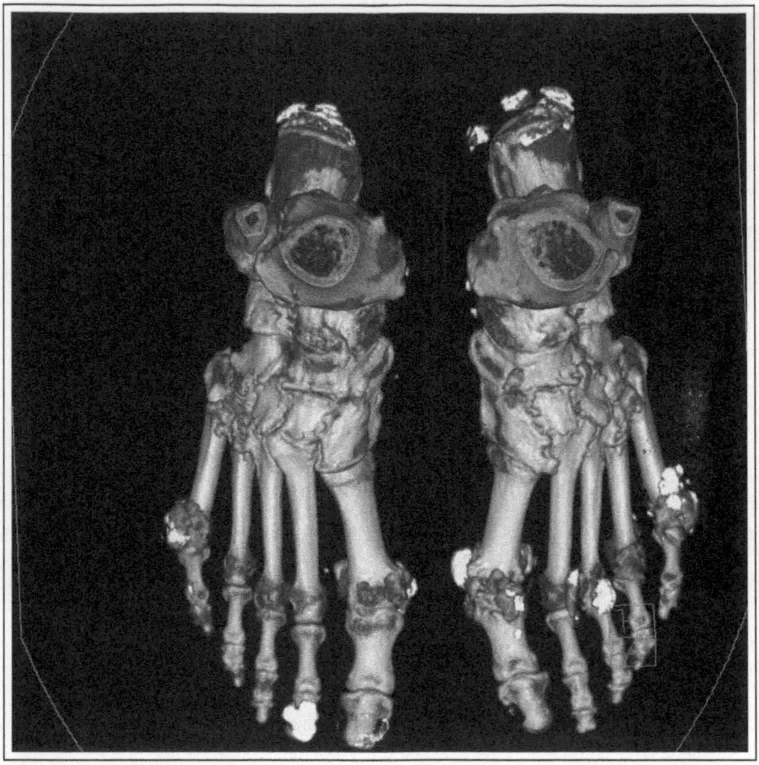

Figure 7.6 Dual energy CT scan in a patient with tophaceous gout. Note the characteristic sites of urate deposition including the first metatarsophalangeal joint and Achilles tendon. (See colour version on inside cover.)

of gout (Choi et al. 2009) (Figure 7.6). In addition to detecting urate deposits, DECT captures other features of gout as described for conventional CT, including the soft tissue response within the tophus and bone disease.

The diagnostic accuracy of DECT has been analyzed in a systematic review and meta-analysis using crystal-proven gout as the diagnostic gold standard (Ogdie et al. 2014). The pooled sensitivity for DECT was 87% and the pooled specificity was 84%. It should be noted that only three studies with a total of 92 patients met inclusion criteria for this meta-analysis. Most of the patients had long-standing disease, and DECT is not typically required for gout diagnosis in this context.

The role of DECT for diagnosis of gout early in disease has not been formally reported. However, there are some suggestions that this modality may not function so well in this situation. In a small study of patients with acute gout, only 50% of patients with the first episode of gout had evidence of urate deposits on DECT (Manger et al. 2012). Furthermore, in a prospective diagnostic study of DECT, false negative results were observed in 30% of patients with acute podagra and no prior episodes of joint pain (Bongartz et al. 2014). Artefact, particularly at the nail bed and heel pads, requires careful exclusion (Mallinson et al. 2014). Thus, the sensitivity of this modality may be much lower in the context of early disease. The lower sensitivity may be explained by the observation that DECT can identify 'dense' urate deposits (with at least 15–20 vol% urate), but that deposits with lower urate volumes may not be detected on the colour-coded DECT images (Melzer et al. 2014).

DECT allows detection of greater urate deposition than is clinically apparent in people with tophaceous gout (Choi et al. 2009). DECT is able to identify urate crystal deposition both in joints and in subcutaneous sites and soft tissue structures such as tendons and ligaments (Dalbeth et al. 2013). Automated volume assessment software allows rapid measurement of urate crystal burden at scanned sites, without the need for time-consuming manual outlining methods used for conventional CT and MRI volume measurements. This method of volume assessment has very high reproducibility (inter-reader intraclass correlation coefficients typically ≥0.95) (Choi et al. 2012). It should be noted that DECT detects only urate deposits, and not the soft tissue component of the tophus. Therefore, analysis of clinically apparent tophi with similar physical characteristics shows large variation in the amount of urate crystal deposition within these lesions (Dalbeth et al. 2012b).

DECT urate deposits can reduce in response to intensive urate-lowering therapy; a recent report has compared DECT scans in people before and after treatment with pegloticase (Araujo et al. 2015). Pegloticase responders (with reduction of serum urate level below 0.36 mmol/L [6 mg/dL] during at least 80% of the treatment time), were virtually cleared of urate deposition (−94.8%) after approximately three months of treatment. It is unknown whether less intensive urate-lowering therapy leads to such profound reductions in DECT urate deposition.

As with conventional CT, the use of ionizing radiation and high cost of DECT may limit the use of this modality in clinical practice. A further issue is that dual source, dual energy scanners with gout software are not widely available.

References

Araujo EG, et al. (2015). Tophus resolution with pegloticase: a prospective dual-energy CT study. *RMD Open*, 1(1), e000075. doi:10.1136/rmdopen-2015-000075

Bloch C, Hermann G, Yu TF (1980). A radiologic reevaluation of gout: a study of 2,000 patients. *AJR American Journal of Roentgenology*, 134(4), 781–7.

Bongartz T, et al. (2014). Dual-energy CT for the diagnosis of gout: an accuracy and diagnostic yield study. *Annals of the Rheumatic Diseases* (early online).

Choi HK, et al. (2009). Dual energy computed tomography in tophaceous gout. *Annals of the Rheumatic Diseases*, 68(10), 1609–12.

Choi HK, et al. (2012). Dual energy CT in gout: a prospective validation study. *Annals of the Rheumatic Diseases*, 71(9), 1466–71.

Cimmino MA, et al. (2011). MRI synovitis and bone lesions are common in acute gouty arthritis of the wrist even during the first attack. *Annals of the Rheumatic Diseases*, 70(12), 2238–9.

Dalbeth N, et al. (2007a). Validation of a radiographic damage index in chronic gout *Arthritis & Rheumatism*, 57(6), 1067–73.

Dalbeth N, et al. (2012a), Characterization of new bone formation in gout: a quantitative site-by-site analysis using plain radiography and computed tomography. *Arthritis Research & Therapy*, 14(4), R165.

Dalbeth N, et al. (2014). Exploratory study of radiographic change in patients with tophaceous gout treated with intensive urate-lowering therapy. *Arthritis Care & Research (Hoboken)*, 66(1), 82–5.

Dalbeth N, et al. (2007b). Computed tomography measurement of tophus volume: comparison with physical measurement. *Arthritis & Rheumatism*, 57(3), 461–5.

Dalbeth N, et al. (2013). Tendon involvement in the feet of patients with gout: a dual-energy CT study. *Annals of the Rheumatic Diseases*, 72(9), 1545–8.

Dalbeth N, et al. (2009). Mechanisms of bone erosion in gout: a quantitative analysis using plain radiography and computed tomography. *Annals of the Rheumatic Diseases*, 68(8), 1290–5.

Dalbeth N, et al. (2012b), Assessment of tophus size: a comparison between physical measurement methods and dual-energy computed tomography scanning. *Journal of Clinical Rheumatology*, 18(1), 23–7.

Dalbeth N, et al. (2015). A multicenter randomized double-blind phase 2 study to evaluate the effect of febuxostat versus placebo on joint damage in hyperuricemic subjects with early gout. Presented at the European League Against Rheumatism annual scientific meeting (Rome).

Gerster JC, et al. (1996). Computed tomography of the knee joint as an indicator of intraarticular tophi in gout. *Arthritis & Rheumatism*, 39(8), 1406–9.

Graser A, et al. (2008). Dual energy CT characterization of urinary calculi: initial in vitro and clinical experience. *Investigative Radiology*, 43(2), 112–9.

Grassi W, et al. (2006). 'Crystal clear'-sonographic assessment of gout and calcium pyrophosphate deposition disease. *Seminars in Arthritis & Rheumatism*, 36(3), 197–202.

Konatalapalli RM, et al. (2012). Correlates of axial gout: a cross-sectional study. *Journal of Rheumatology*, 39(7), 1445–1449.

Mallinson PI, et al. (2014). Artifacts in dual-energy CT gout protocol: a review of 50 suspected cases with an artifact identification guide. *AJR American Journal of Roentgenology*, 203(1), W103–9.

Manger B, et al. (2012). Detection of periarticular urate deposits with dual energy CT in patients with acute gouty arthritis. *Annals of the Rheumatic Diseases*, 71(3), 470–2.

McQueen FM, et al. (2014). Bone erosions in patients with chronic gouty arthropathy are associated with tophi but not bone oedema or synovitis: new insights from a 3 T MRI study. *Rheumatology (Oxford)*, 53(1), 95–103.

Melzer R, et al. (2014). Gout tophus detection-a comparison of dual-energy CT (DECT) and histology. *Seminars in Arthritis & Rheumatism*, 43(5), 662–5.

Naredo E, et al. (2014). Ultrasound-detected musculoskeletal urate crystal deposition: which joints and what findings should be assessed for diagnosing gout? *Annals of the Rheumatic Diseases*, 73(8), 1522–8.

Neogi T, et al. (2015). 2015 gout classification criteria: an American College of Rheumatology/European League Against Rheumatism collaborative initiative. *Arthritis & Rheumatology*, 67(10), 2557–2568.

Nicolaou S, et al. (2010). Dual-energy CT as a potential new diagnostic tool in the management of gout in the acute setting. *AJR American Journal of Roentgenology*, 194(4), 1072–8.

Ogdie A, et al. (2014). Imaging modalities for the classification of gout: systematic literature review and meta-analysis. *Annals of the Rheumatic Diseases*. doi:10.1136/annrheumdis-2014-205431

Ogdie A, et al. (2015). Value of musculoskeletal ultrasound for the diagnosis of gout in a large multi-center study: comparison with monosodium urate crystal analysis. Presented at the American College of Rheumatology annual scientific meeting (San Francisco, CA).

Perez-Ruiz F, Martin I, Canteli B (2007). Ultrasonographic measurement of tophi as an outcome measure for chronic gout. *Journal of Rheumatology*, 34(9), 1888–93.

Pineda C, et al. (2011). Joint and tendon subclinical involvement suggestive of gouty arthritis in asymptomatic hyperuricemia: an ultrasound controlled study. *Arthritis Research & Therapy*, 13(1), R4.

Poh YJ, et al. (2011). Magnetic resonance imaging bone edema is not a major feature of gout unless there is concomitant osteomyelitis: 10-year findings from a high-prevalence population. *Journal of Rheumatology*, 38(11), 2475–81.

Popovich I, et al. (2014). Exploring cartilage damage in gout using 3-T MRI: distribution and associations with joint inflammation and tophus deposition. *Skeletal Radiology*, 43(7), 917–24.

Popp JD, Bidgood WD, Jr, Edwards NL (1996). Magnetic resonance imaging of tophaceous gout in the hands and wrists. *Seminars in Arthritis & Rheumatism*, 25(4), 282–9.

Thiele RG and Schlesinger N (2007). Diagnosis of gout by ultrasound. *Rheumatology (Oxford)*, 46 (7), 1116–21.

Yu JS, et al. (1997). MR imaging of tophaceous gout. *AJR American Journal of Roentgenology*, 168(2), 523–7.

Chapter 8

Principles of gout management

Key points

- The main goal of therapy is to achieve 'remission'—the absence of gout attacks and tophi.
- A sustained reduction in serum urate is critical to the long-term management of gout and will ultimately result in cessation of gout attacks and resolution of tophi.
- Target serum urate is <0.36 mmol/L for everyone, although a lower target of <0.30 mmol/L may be required for those with severe tophaceous disease.
- Patient and physician education about the causes and effective management of gout are required to improve adherence to therapy and long-term outcomes.

The management of gout can be divided into five key areas: (1) making an accurate diagnosis; (2) long-term preventative therapy through adequate urate lowering; (3) adequate prophylaxis against acute attacks during the introduction of urate-lowering therapy; (4) effective therapy of acute attacks; and (5) appropriate screening and management of associated co-morbidities. Management includes both pharmacological and non-pharmacological aspects. Patient education is critical to successful management in each of the five key areas. This chapter will discuss the broad management concepts with diagnosis, specific pharmacological treatment of acute gout and urate-lowering therapy, as well as screening for co-morbidities discussed in detail in other elsewhere in this volume (Chapters 9–11).

8.1 Goal of therapy and treatment targets

The main goal of therapy is to achieve 'remission'; that is, the absence of gout attacks and tophi. A sustained reduction in serum urate below saturation concentrations leads to dissolution of monosodium urate (MSU) crystals, which ultimately results in cessation of gout attacks and resolution of tophi.

There are currently two recommended serum urate targets: <0.36 mmol/L and <0.30 mmol/L. The American College of Rheumatology (ACR) and European League Against Rheumatism (EULAR) guidelines recommend a minimum serum urate <0.36 mmol/L, while the British Society for Rheumatology (BSR) guidelines recommend <0.30 mmol/L. The ACR guidelines acknowledge a lower target may be required in those with severe or tophaceous disease. These serum urate targets are based on evidence that gout attacks and urate stores deplete with sustained reduction in serum urate <0.36 mmol/L (Li-Yu et al. 2001; Shoji et al. 2004). A study examining the relationship between tophus size and serum urate during urate-lowering therapy reported a reduction in tophus size of 0.53 ± 0.59 mm/month in patients with a mean serum urate of 0.36–0.42 mmol/L, 0.77 ± 0.41 mm/month in those with a mean serum urate of 0.30–0.36 mmol/L, 0.99 ± 0.50 mm/month in those with serum urate 0.24–0.30 mmol/L, and 1.52 ± 0.67 mm/month in those with mean serum urate

≤0.24 mmol/L. In addition, there was a linear relationship between mean serum urate and speed of tophus size reduction ($r = -0.62$; $r^2 = 0.48$; $p < 0.05$) (Perez-Ruiz et al. 2002). The lower the serum urate, the faster the reduction in tophus size; hence consideration should be given to a lower target in this group of patients. Achieving target serum urate has also been associated with lower medical costs (Halpern et al. 2009).

Concerns have been raised about the potential for harm with sustained reduction in serum urate. In observational studies, low serum urate levels have been associated with poor outcomes in acute ischaemic stroke (Wu et al. 2014), lower bone mineral density (Nabipour et al. 2011), poor cognitive function (Molshatzki et al. 2015), Parkinson's disease (Shen and Ji 2013), loss of kidney function (Kanda et al. 2015), and all-cause and cardiovascular mortality (Kuo et al. 2013). Further research is required to determine the optimal target serum urate and duration at target at different stages of hyperuricaemia and gout. Whether a higher serum urate can maintain 'remission' once this state has been achieved and sustained also needs to be determined.

8.2 Barriers to successful management of gout

The main barriers to optimal patient care in gout are low adherence with urate-lowering therapy, and poor patient and physician understanding of the disease and its management. A recent systematic review of adherence in gout revealed only 10–46% of patients adhere to gout treatments (De Vera et al. 2014). Gout has the lowest patient medication adherence rate among chronic diseases (Briesacher et al. 2008), and adherence with non-pharmacological management is likely even lower (Reach 2011). A number of patient variables have been associated with lower adherence rates, including younger age, absence of tophi, gout flares, ethnicity, and allopurinol dose escalation (De Vera et al. 2014). Other patient-identified barriers to urate-lowering therapy adherence include adverse effects, doubts about effectiveness, cost, concern about drug interactions, and forgetfulness (Singh 2014).

Insufficient patient and physician understanding of the disease itself and the aims and modalities of treatment is a primary reason for poor management and poor clinical outcomes. The greater patients' understanding of their illness, the more likely they are to adhere to urate-lowering therapy (Dalbeth et al. 2011). Thus, ensuring patient understanding is critical in gout management, and patient education is included in key management guidelines (Khanna et al. 2012a; W. Zhang et al. 2006). However, few patients recall clear explanations of gout or lifestyle advice (Roddy et al. 2007). This may be at least in part due to negative stereotypes about gout and a lack of understanding of the underlying cause of gout and its management by doctors (Harrold et al. 2013; Spencer et al. 2012). Compounding this is variability and often poor information in patient resources on gout. Many resources are written well above the average reading level, and key content is absent from many resources (Johnston et al. 2015; Robinson and Schumacher 2013). For example, in one study of 30 different resources from six countries, less than 50% of resources mention the target serum urate and only 30% advised continuation of urate-lowering therapy during acute gout attacks (Figure 8.1) (Johnston et al. 2015).

When appropriate education and monitoring are provided, evidence from both nurse-led and pharmacist-led programmes suggests that outcomes improve (Goldfien et al. 2014; Rees et al. 2013). Education of health care providers about prescription and dosing of urate-lowering therapies is also required (Dalbeth et al. 2012a).

8.3 Management of gout flares

Treatment of acute gout flares is directed at suppression of the inflammatory response to MSU crystals. Treatment should be commenced as early as possible after the onset of

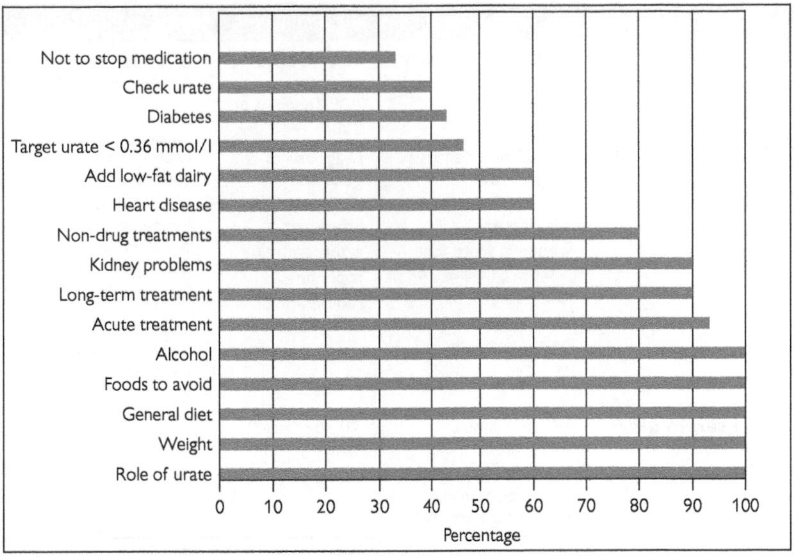

Figure 8.1 Percentage of patient educational resources that cover important messages in gout treatment. Source data from Johnston, ME, et al. (2015), 'Patient Information about Gout: An International Review of Existing Educational Resources', J Rheumatol, 42 (6), 975-8.

the gout attack and preferably within 24 hours after onset. Patients should be educated on self-management of gout flare and have a supply of the preferred treatment agent on hand so they can initiate treatment without the need to see a health care professional during an acute flare. Non-pharmacological therapy of acute gout includes rest and topical ice application of the affected joint (Schlesinger et al. 2002).

The three readily available agents for treatment of acute gout are non-steroidal anti-inflammatories, colchicine, and corticosteroids. More recently, interleukin-1 inhibitors have been used in the management of acute gout, but they are not widely approved and their use is limited by cost. The choice of agent is dictated by the patient's co-morbidities and concomitant medications. Where the attack is severe and/or polyarticular, combination therapy such as NSAID and colchicine, or corticosteroids plus colchicine may be appropriate. Treatment should be continued until the attack has fully settled and in the case of oral corticosteroids should then be tapered over 7–10 days as rebound flares may occur if treatment is discontinued to early. Should the gout flare not settle as expected, alternative diagnoses should be considered, particularly septic arthritis, which can co-exist with gout. It is also important to educate patients that urate-lowering therapy should not be stopped during acute gout attacks.

8.4 Urate-lowering therapy: indications and therapeutic options

The key indications for urate-lowering therapy are a diagnosis of gout and either recurrent attacks or presence of tophi. There are subtle variations in other indications as outlined in Table 8.1. Urate-lowering therapy is not currently indicated in asymptomatic hyperuricaemia or in hyperuricaemia associated with renal or cardiac disease but without symptomatic gout.

Table 8.1 Summary comparison of international guidelines for management of gout

	ACR 2012 guidelines (Khanna et al. 2012a)	EULAR 2006 guidelines (W. Zhang et al. 2006)	BSR 2007 guidelines (Jordan et al. 2007)
Indications for ULT	Established diagnosis of gout ***and*** tophi by exam or imaging ***or*** frequent acute gout attacks (≥2/year) ***or*** CKD stage 2 or worse ***or*** past urolithiasis	Diagnosis of gout ***and*** recurrent acute attacks ***or*** arthropathy ***or*** tophi ***or*** radiographic changes of gout	Diagnosis of gout ***and*** second attack, or further attacks occur within 1 yr ***or*** tophi ***or*** renal insufficiency ***or*** uric acid stones ***or*** need to continue treatment with diuretics
Target serum urate (SU)	<0.36 mmol/L minimum For severe or tophaceous disease may need <0.30 mmol/L	<0.36 mmol/L for all	<0.30 mmol/L for all
Lifestyle	Yes	Yes	Yes
Patient education	Yes	Yes	Not specifically mentioned
Co-morbidity screening	Yes	Yes	Yes
Urate-lowering therapy	First-line: allopurinol or febuxostat Second-line: uricosuric Third-line: pegloticase	First-line: allopurinol Second-line: uricosuric	First-line: allopurinol Second-line: uricosuric
Acute gout pharmacologic treatment	First-line: NSAID, colchicine, or corticosteroid	First-line: NSAID or colchicine Second-line: corticosteroid	Not ranked—consider NSAID, colchicine, or corticosteroid
Acute gout non-pharmacologic measures	Ice		Rest and elevate joint Bed cage Ice
Prophylaxis during ULT initiation	Yes First-line: colchicine Second-line: NSAID Duration: the greatest of at least 6 months or 3 months after achieving target SU if no tophi or 6 months after achieving target if tophi present	Yes Colchicine or NSAID No comment on duration	Yes First-line: colchicine for up to 6 months Second-line: NSAID, but duration should be limited to 6 weeks

Three classes of urate-lowering therapy are available: (a) xanthine oxidase inhibitors, which prevent urate production (e.g. allopurinol, febuxostat); (b) uricosurics, which normalize renal uric acid excretion (e.g. probenecid, benzbromarone); and (c) recombinant uricases, which degrade urate (e.g. pegloticase).. A xanthine oxidase inhibitor is recommended as the first-line urate-lowering therapy, although febuxostat is not specifically mentioned in the currently published 2006 EULAR or BSR guidelines as it was introduced after these recommendations were published. Uricosuric agents are considered second-line therapy. They should replace a xanthine oxidase inhibitor if neither is tolerated, or be added to a xanthine oxidase inhibitor if target urate is not achieved with monotherapy. Pegloticase is a third-line treatment reserved for those patients with severe, refractory disease who have failed therapy with a xanthine oxidase inhibitor in combination with a uricosuric at maximum appropriate doses.

8.5 Anti-inflammatory prophylaxis

There is a high rate of gout flares during initiation of urate-lowering therapy; thus anti-inflammatory prophylaxis against gout flares is recommended during this high-risk period (typically at least three months, but longer periods may be beneficial, particularly for patients with high urate crystal load). All the current guidelines recommended colchicine or NSAID for anti-inflammatory prophylaxis, but there is no consensus on the duration of treatment (Table 8.1).

8.6 Lifestyle advice

The role of diet in the aetiology and management of gout is portrayed in historical caricatures of gout. The association between rich foods and alcohol has contributed to the stigma of gout. The renewed interest in gout over the past decade has seen changes to the dietary and lifestyle advice for gout patients. However, there remains variation and conflicting advice about what foods to avoid and what to encourage in patients with gout (Johnston et al. 2015). The 2012 ACR guidelines are the most up-to-date and comprehensive with respect to diet (Table 8.2) (Khanna et al. 2012a). Dietary and/or lifestyle modifications alone are generally insufficient to achieve target serum urate. Furthermore, dietary modification is difficult to sustain in the long term, and even comprehensive education about the role of diet has been shown to have no effect on serum urate in patients on urate-lowering therapy (Holland and McGill 2015). Therefore, lifestyle advice should be considered an adjunct to urate-lowering medications.

The traditional dietary advice for patients with gout entails limiting or avoiding foods and drinks that contain higher amounts of purines or are thought to precipitate acute attacks of gout. These may include meat, seafood, beer and wine, and legumes. Such diets are frequently high in saturated fats and carbohydrates, which may add to the risk of metabolic syndrome.

More recently there has been interest in other dietary components or supplements. Vitamin C (ascorbic acid) is an important vitamin that can be obtained only through dietary intake. It is water-soluble and is not stored within the body. Therefore the diet must contain vitamin C to maintain the ascorbic acid pool. Dietary sources of ascorbic acid include fresh fruits and vegetables; in particular, citrus fruits and green leafy vegetables, such as broccoli. Compared with no supplementation, supplementation of the diet with vitamin C 1.0–1.5 g daily has been reported to reduce the risk of gout (OR = 0.66, 95% CI [0.49, 0.88]) (H. Choi et al. 2009). In individuals without gout, vitamin C 500 mg daily has been reported to lower serum urate (mean reduction of −0.03 mmol/L (95% CI [−0.04, −0.02], $P < 0.0001$) (Huang et al. 2005). However, in a small study of patients with gout, vitamin C 500 mg/day for 8 weeks had no clinically significant urate-lowering effect alone or in combination with allopurinol (Stamp et al. 2013).

Table 8.2 Lifestyle recommendations in current gout guidelines			
	ACR 2012 guidelines (Khanna et al. 2012b)	EULAR 2006 guidelines (W. Zhang et al. 2006)	BSR 2007 guidelines (Jordan et al. 2007)
Weight	Weight loss for obese BMI that promotes general health	Weight loss if obese	Weight loss to achieve ideal body weight
Encourage	Low- or non-fat dairy Vegetables	General recommendation that diet core aspect of management No specific dietary advice	Skimmed milk/low-fat dairy Soy beans Cherries
Limit	Serving sizes of beef, lamb, pork, and high-purine seafood Naturally sweet fruit juices Sugar: table sugar, sweetened beverages, desserts Table salt		Red meat and high-protein foods Overall protein intake
Avoid	High-purine organs: liver, kidney, sweetbreads High-fructose corn syrup–sweetened sodas, beverages, or foods		Liver, kidneys, shellfish, and yeast extracts
Water	Stay well hydrated	No comment	If history of urolithiasis, >2 litres daily and consider alkalinization Avoid dehydration
Alcohol	≤2 servings daily (men) and ≤1 serving daily (women) Any alcohol, if frequent attacks or advanced gout under poor control	Reduce, especially beer	<21 units/week (men) and <14 units/week (women)At least 3 alcohol-free days/week Avoid beer, stout, port, and similar fortified wines

Cherries and tart cherry concentrate have also been reported to reduce serum urate and prevent gout flares (Jacob et al. 2003; Schlesinger and Schlesinger 2012; Y. Zhang et al. 2012). The mechanisms of action of cherries remains unclear and is likely multifactorial. Cherry products contain high levels of anthocyanins which have a number of anti-inflammatory and anti-oxidant effects, including inhibition of cyclo-oxygenase and scavenging of nitric oxide radicals (Seeram et al. 2001; van Acker et al. 1995; Wang et al. 1999).

Fructose, which is found in corn syrup, sugar-sweetened soft drinks, and fruit juices, has been associated with both hyperuricaemia and gout (H. Choi and Curhan 2008; J. Choi et al. 2008). Furthermore, urate and fructose share a common transporter within the kidney (*SLC2A9*) (Vitart et al. 2008), which may be influenced by dietary intake of sugars derived from sugar-sweetened beverages (Batt et al. 2014). Avoidance of fructose is therefore recommended in patients with gout. Low-fat dairy products also have been inversely associated with serum urate (H. Choi et al. 2005), and skim milk may reduce gout flares (Dalbeth et al. 2012b).

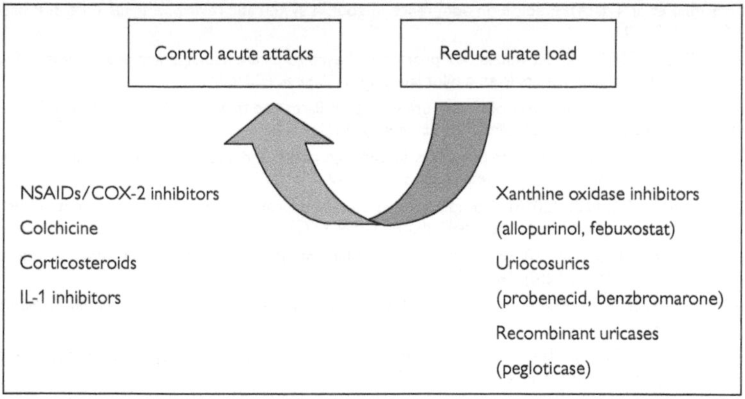

Figure 8.2 Principles of gout management.

8.7 **Summary**

In conclusion, effective urate lowering will lead to dissolution of urate crystals, cessation of acute attacks, and resolution of tophi (Figure 8.2). Patient and physician education about the causes and effective management of gout are required to improve adherence to therapy and long-term outcomes. There are effective therapies for acute gout attacks, and patients should have an action plan to rapidly self-manage flares. Ultimately, dietary and lifestyle modifications have a limited role in urate lowering.

References

Batt C, et al. (2014). Sugar-sweetened beverage consumption: a risk factor for prevalent gout with SLC2A9 genotypespecific effects on serum urate and risk of gout. *Annals of the Rheumatic Diseases*, 73(12), 2101–6.

Briesacher BA, et al. (2008). Comparison of drug adherence rates among patients with seven different medical conditions. *Pharmacotherapy*, 28(4), 437–43.

Choi HK and Curhan G (2008). Soft drinks, fructose consumption, and the risk of gout in men: prospective cohort study. *BMJ*, 336, 309–12.

Choi HK, Liu S, Curhan G (2005). Intake of purine-rich foods, protein and dairy products and relationship to serum levels of uric acid. *Arthritis & Rheumatism*, 52(1), 283–9.

Choi HK, Gao X, Curhan G (2009). Vitamin C intake and the risk of gout in men: a prospective study. *Archives of Internal Medicine*, 169(5), 502–07.

Choi JWJ, et al. (2008). Sugar-sweetened soft drinks, diet soft drinks and serum uric acid level: The Third National Health and Nutrition Examination Survey. *Arthritis Care & Research*, 59(1), 109–16.

Dalbeth N, et al. (2011). Illness perceptions in patients with gout and the relationship with progression of musculoskeletal disease. *Arthritis Care & Research*, 63(11), 1605–12.

Dalbeth N, et al. (2012a). Prescription and dosing of urate-lowering therapy, rather than patient behaviours, are the key modifiable factors associated with targeting serum urate in gout. *BMC Musculoskeletal Disorders*, 13, 174.

Dalbeth N, et al. (2012b). Effects of skim milk powder enriched with glycomacropeptide and G600 milk fat extract on frequency of gout flares: a proof-of-concept randomised controlled trial. *Annals of the Rheumatic Diseases*, 71, 929–34.

De Vera MA, et al. (2014). Medication adherence in gout: a systematic review. *Arthritis Care & Research*, 66(10), 1551–9.

Goldfien RD, et al. (2014). Effectiveness of a pharmacist-based gout care management programme in a large integrated health plan: results from a pilot study. *BMJ Open*, 4, e003627.

Halpern R, et al. (2009). The effect of serum urate on gout flares and their associated costs: an administrative claims analysis. *Journal of Clinical Rheumatology*, 15(1), 3–7.

Harrold LR, et al. (2013). Primary care providers' knowledge, beliefs and treatment practices for gout: results of a physician questionnaire. *Rheumatology*, 52, 1623–9.

Holland R and McGill NW (2015). Comprehensive dietary education in treated gout patients does not further improve serum urate. *Internal Medicine Journal*, 45(2), 189–94.

Huang H-Y, et al. (2005). The effects of vitamin C supplementation on serum concentrations of uric acid. *Arthritis & Rheumatism*, 52(6), 1843–7.

Jacob RA, et al. (2003). Consumption of cherries lowers plasma urate in healthy women. *Journal of Nutrition*, 13, 1826–9.

Johnston ME, et al. (2015). Patient information about gout: an international review of existing educational resources. *Journal of Rheumatology*, 42(6), 975–8.

Jordan KM, et al. (2007). British Society for Rheumatology and British Health Professionals in Rheumatology guideline for the management of gout. *Rheumatology*, 46(8), 1372–4.

Kanda E, et al. (2015). Uric acid level has a U-shaped association with loss of kidney function in healthy people: a prospective cohort study. *PLoS One*, 10(2), e0118031.

Khanna D, et al. (2012a). 2012 American College of Rheumatology Guidelines for the Management of Gout. Part 1: Systematic nonpharmacologic and pharmacologic therapeutic approaches to hyperuricaemia. *Arthritis Care & Research*, 64(10), 1431–46.

Khanna D, et al. (2012b). 2012 American College of Rheumatology Guidelines for the Management of Gout. Part 2: Therapy and antiinflammatory prophylaxis of acute gouty arthritis. *Arthritis Care & Research*, 64(10), 1447–61.

Kuo C-F, et al. (2013). Significance of serum uric acid levels on the risk of all-cause and cardiovascular mortality. *Rheumatology*, 52, 127–34.

Li-Yu J, et al. (2001). Treatment of chronic gout: can we determine when urate stores are depleted enough to prevent attacks of gout? *Journal of Rheumatology*, 28, 577–80.

Molshatzki N, et al. (2015). Serum uric acid and subsequent cognitive performance in patients with pre-existing cardiovascular disease. *PLoS One*. doi:10.1371/journal.pone.0120862

Nabipour I, et al. (2011). Serum uric acid is associated with bone health in older men: a cross-sectional population-based study. *Journal of Bone and Mineral Research*, 26(5), 955–64.

Perez-Ruiz F, et al. (2002). Effect of urate-lowering therapy on the velocity of size reduction of tophi in chronic gout. *Arthritis Care & Research*, 47(4), 356–60.

Reach G (2011). Treatment adherence in patients with gout. *Joint Bone Spine*, 78(5), 456–9.

Rees F, Jenkins W, Doherty M (2013). Patients with gout adhere to curative treatment if informed appropriately: proof-of-concept observational study. *Annals of the Rheumatic Diseases*, 72(6), 826–30.

Robinson PC and Schumacher HR (2013). A qualitative and quantitative analysis of the characteristics of gout patient education resources. *Clinical Rheumatology*, 32, 771–8.

Roddy E, Zhang W, Doherty M (2007). Concordance of the management of chronic gout in a UK primary care population with the EULAR gout recommendations. *Annals of the Rheumatic Diseases*, 66, 1311–5.

Schlesinger N and Schlesinger M (2012). Pilot studies of cherry juice concentrate for gout flare prophylaxis. *Journal of Arthritis*, 1(1).

Schlesinger N, et al. (2002). Local ice therapy during bouts of acute gouty arthritis. *Journal of Rheumatology*, 29, 331–4.

Seeram NP, et al.(2001). Cyclooxygenase inhibitory and antioxidant cyanidin glycosides in cherries and berries. *Phytomedicine*, 8(5), 362–9.

Shen L and Ji HF (2013). Low uric acid levels in patients with Parkinson's disease: evidence from meta-analysis. *BMJ Open*, 3, e003620.

Shoji A, Yamanaka H, Kamatani N (2004). A retrospective study of the relationship between serum urate level and recurrent attacks of gouty arthritis: evidence for reduction of recurrent gouty arthritis with antihyperuricaemic therapy. *Arthritis Care & Research*, 51(3), 321–5.

Singh JA (2014). Facilitators and barriers to adherence to urate-lowering therapy in African-Americans with gout: a qualitative study. *Arthritis Research & Therapy*, 16, R82.

Spencer K, Carr AC, Doherty M (2012). Patient and provider barriers to effective management of gout in general practice: a qualitative study. *Annals of the Rheumatic Diseases*, 71, 1490–5.

Stamp LK, et al. (2013). Clinically insignificant effect of supplemental vitamin C on serum urate in patients with gout; a pilot randomised controlled trial. *Arthritis & Rheumatism*, 65(6), 1636–42.

Vanacker SABE, et al. (1995). Flavonoids as scavengers of nitric oxide radical. *Biochemical and Biophysical Research Communications*, 214(3), 755–9.

Vitart V, et al. (2008). SLC2A9 is a newly identified urate transporter influencing serum urate concentration, urate excretion and gout. *Nature Genetics*, 40, 437–42.

Wang H, et al. (1999). Novel antioxidant compounds from tart cherries (Prunus cerasus). *Journal of Natural Products*, 62 (1), 86–8.

Wu H, et al. (2014). Decreased uric acid levels correlate with poor outcomes in acute ischemic stroke patients, but not in cerebral hemorrhage patients. *Journal of Stroke and Cerebrovascular Diseases*, 23(3), 469–75.

Zhang W, et al. (2006). EULAR evidence based recommendations for gout. Part II: Management. Report of a task force of the EULAR Standing Committee for International Clinical Studies Including Therapeutics (ESCISIT). *Annals of the Rheumatic Diseases*, 65 (10), 1312–24.

Zhang Y, et al. (2012). Cherry consumption and decreased risk of recurrent gout attacks. *Arthritis & Rheumatism*, 64(12), 4004–11.

Chapter 9

Urate-lowering therapy agents

Key points

- Xanthine oxidase inhibitors (allopurinol or febuxostat) a considered first-line urate-lowering therapy.
- Combination therapy with uricosuric agents may be required.
- The choice of urate-lowering therapy is dictated by co-morbidities, particularly renal and hepatic impairment.
- Appropriate monitoring for drug adverse effects as well as serum urate to ensure targets are achieved is required.

Urate-lowering therapy is critical in the management of gout. Serum urate can be lowered by (a) inhibition of urate production through use of xanthine oxidase inhibitors, such as allopurinol and febuxostat; (b) normalization of renal uric acid excretion with the use of selective uric acid resorption inhibitors, such as probenecid and benzbromarone; and (c) dissolution of urate though use of recombinant uricases, such as pegloticase (Figure 9.1).

Xanthine oxidase inhibition is recommended as first-line therapy (Khanna et al. 2012; Sivera et al. 2014). In patients who fail to achieve target serum urate, combination therapy with a xanthine oxidase inhibitor and a uricosuric may be appropriate. Recombinant uricases are generally reserved for the individuals with a high urate burden and refractory disease, although studies are ongoing to determine their optimal administration. This chapter will review the urate-lowering therapies currently available.

9.1 Allopurinol

Allopurinol is the most commonly used urate-lowering therapy. Despite the introduction of newer agents, it is likely to remain a first-line agent as it is cheap and readily available.

9.1.1 Mechanism of action

Allopurinol is rapidly metabolized to its active metabolite oxypurinol. Both allopurinol and oxypurinol inhibit xanthine oxidase, thereby reducing urate production. Oxypurinol is responsible for the majority of xanthine oxidase inhibition due to its longer half-life and much stronger binding to the reduced form of xanthine oxidase.

9.1.2 Clinical pharmacology

Allopurinol is readily absorbed from the gastrointestinal tract. The majority (~80%) of allopurinol is metabolized to oxypurinol by aldehyde oxidase and to a lesser extent xanthine oxidase, while ~10% is metabolized to allopurinol-1′-riboside. The half-life of allopurinol is ~1 hour. Oxypurinol is largely eliminated unchanged via the kidneys, and its half-life is dependent on renal function. In patients with normal renal function, half-life is ~23 hours, while virtually no oxypurinol is excreted in anuric patients (Hande et al. 1984).

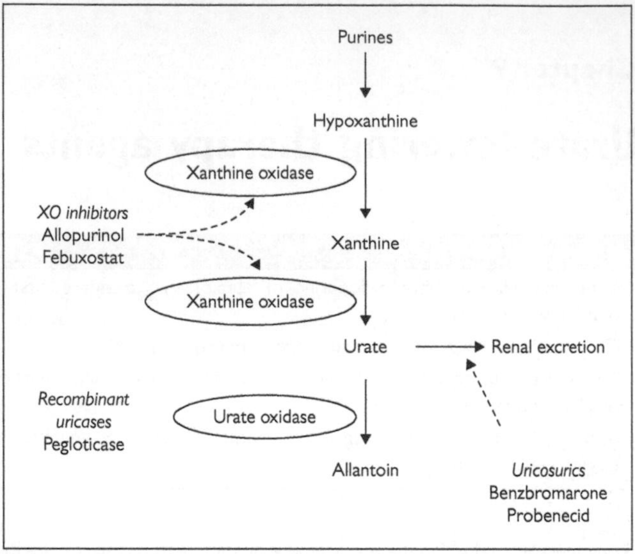

Figure 9.1 Site of action of urate-lowering therapies.

9.1.3 **Allopurinol dosing**

Allopurinol dosing remains controversial, especially in patients with renal impairment. The observed association between allopurinol dose, renal impairment, and allopurinol hypersensitivity syndrome (AHS) led to the suggestion that allopurinol dose should be reduced in the setting of renal impairment in order to minimize the risk of this serious adverse event (Hande et al. 1984). This renal-based dosing has led to a general reluctance—even in patients with normal renal function—to use more than 300 mg daily, and many patients who receive allopurinol do not achieve target serum urate (Annemans et al. 2008; Dalbeth et al. 2006; Day et al. 1988). Recent evidence suggests that the starting dose of allopurinol, but not the maintenance dose, is associated with AHS (Stamp et al. 2012b). Starting at low dose (e.g. allopurinol 1.5 mg per mL/min eGFR daily) is suggested as reasonable to minimize the risk of AHS (Stamp et al. 2012b).

This is consistent with the American College of Rheumatology (ACR) guidelines, which recommend that no patient start on more than 100 mg daily, and in those with creatinine clearance (CrCL) <60 mL/min, the starting dose should be 50 mg daily (Khanna et al. 2012). The ACR guidelines also recommend gradual allopurinol dose increase (with appropriate patient education and monitoring in those who tolerate it) in order to achieve target serum urate.

Evidence for such an approach is growing. Doubling the dose of allopurinol from 300 to 600 mg daily in patients with CrCL >50 mL/min resulted in 78% of patients achieving target serum urate without any additional adverse effects (Reinders et al. 2009b). In our small pilot study, a more structured allopurinol dose-escalation strategy was safe and effective, with 88.8% of patients achieving the target serum urate of <0.36 mmol/L at 12 months when the allopurinol dose was increased above the CrCL-based dose (Stamp et al. 2011b). A larger study of the safety and efficacy of this approach is currently under way (Australian New Zealand Clinical Trials Registry Number 12611000845932).

9.1.4 **Drug interactions**

One of the most important interactions is that between allopurinol and azathioprine. The active metabolite of azathioprine, 6-mercaptopurine, is partly inactivated by xanthine oxidase. Inhibition of xanthine oxidase by allopurinol can therefore result in increased 6-mercaptopurine concentrations and pancytopenia (Venkat Raman et al. 1990). This is of particular relevance for patients with renal transplants where azathioprine use is common, as is gout (Stamp et al. 2006). The safest approach is to avoid the allopurinol/azathioprine combination. If the combination must be used, the dose of both allopurinol and azathioprine should be reduced, and careful monitoring is required.

There is also a clinically significant interaction between allopurinol and furosemide such that patients on furosemide have higher serum urate concentrations despite higher plasma oxypurinol concentrations (Stamp et al. 2012a). Patients receiving furosemide also require higher doses of allopurinol relative to renal function to achieve the target serum urate (Stamp et al. 2011b). It is important that clinicians regularly review the need for furosemide in patients with gout. Other drug interactions are summarized in Table 9.1.

9.1.5 **Clinical efficacy data**

Allopurinol has specifically been shown to be effective in reducing serum urate, resorption of tophi, and reducing the number of gout flares. Allopurinol is considered a weak urate-lowering therapy. Clinical trials report a reduction in serum urate with allopurinol but only a minority of patients achieve the target serum urate (Becker et al. 2005; Schumacher et al. 2008). However, much of this apparent 'poor efficacy' may be explained by poor adherence (Harrold et al. 2009; Riedel et al. 2004), use of fixed or renal-based allopurinol doses (Dalbeth et al. 2006), or both. As noted, recent evidence suggests that progressive allopurinol dose escalation results in the majority of patients achieving target serum urate (Stamp et al. 2011b). Reduction and eventual cessation of gout flares can be achieved with a sustained reduction in serum urate to <0.36 mmol/L, along with a reduction in the size and number of tophi.

9.1.6 **Adverse effects**

Allopurinol is generally well tolerated. Approximately 2% of patients develop a mild rash (McInnes et al. 1981) and up to 5% stop allopurinol due to adverse events. The most feared adverse effect is AHS. Other severe adverse events have been described, including severe cutaneous adverse reaction (SCAR) and drug reaction with eosinophilia and systemic symptoms (DRESS). These syndromes share clinical characteristics of rash—ranging from a mild maculopapular rash to Stevens Johnson/toxic epidermal necrolysis (SJS/TEN) or exfoliative dermatitis—combined with eosinophilia, leukocytosis, fever, hepatitis, and progressive renal failure.

Allopurinol is the most common cause of SJS/TEN in Europe and Israel (Halevy et al. 2008) and is second most common cause of DRESS (Kardaun et al. 2013). AHS typically occurs early after starting allopurinol, with 90% of cases occurring within 8–9 weeks (Ramasamy et al. 2013). A number of other risk factors for AHS have been identified, which have led to changes in recommendations for the use of allopurinol. HLA-B*58:01 has been associated with AHS, particularly in those of Asian descent. Thus pretreatment testing for HLA-B*58:01 has been recommended in high-risk populations, with avoidance of allopurinol in those who are positive (Hershfield et al. 2013; Khanna et al. 2012). Whether allopurinol 'desensitization' in this high-risk group is safe, while still allowing doses which result in adequate urate lowering, remains to be determined, although preliminary evidence is encouraging (Jung et al. 2015).

Allopurinol starting dose has been reported to be associated with AHS (Stamp et al. 2012b). Impaired renal function is one of the most prominent co-morbidities, occurring in 48% in a

Table 9.1 Important drug interactions to consider when treating patients with gout

	Drugs which may interact	Effect	Clinical consideration/dosing adjustment	Monitoring required
Allopurinol	Furosemide	Increase plasma oxypurinol concentration Increase in SU	May require higher doses of allopurinol to achieve target SU	Creatinine
	Thiazide diuretics	Increase SU	May require higher doses of allopurinol to achieve target SU	
	Azathioprine	Increase 6-mercaptopurine concentrations resulting in myelosuppression	Avoid combination. If must use, reduce azathioprine by 50–75% and use lower dose of allopurinol	Regular full blood count while on combination
	Probenecid	Reduced plasma oxypurinol concentrations Reduced SU		
	Warfarin	May increase anticoagulant effects		Monitor INR
	ACE inhibitors	May increase risk of allergic reaction to allopurinol		Monitor clinically
	Theophylline	Increased serum half-life of theophylline		Monitor serum theophylline concentrations
	Penicillins	May increase risk of skin rash		Monitor clinically
Febuxostat	Azathioprine	Not formally documented but likely increase 6-mercaptopurine concentrations due to XO inhibition resulting in myelosuppression	Avoid combination	
Probenecid	Aspirin high dose	Decreases uricosuric effect		
	Methotrexate	Increases methotrexate concentrations		Monitor for metho-trexate adverse effects

	Pencillins and cephalosporin	Increased antibiotic concentrations		
Benzbromarone	Warfarin	May increase anticoagulant effects	Consider reduction in warfarin dose of 30%	Monitor INR
	Other hepatotoxic drugs	Potential additive effect with respect to hepatotoxicity		Use combinations with caution
	Drugs metabolized by CYP2C9 (e.g. phenytoin, sulfonylureas)	BBR is a moderator inhibitor of CYP2C9, so concentrations of drugs metabolized by this enzyme may increase	Consider dose reduction of drugs metabolized by CYP2C9	Monitor glucose, phenytoin concentrations
	Fluconazole	Increased benzbromarone concentrations	Avoid combination	
	Rifampicin	Induces benzbromarone metabolism	Benzbromarone unlikely to be effective; consider alternative agent	
Pegloticase	No studies			

large case series (Ramasamy et al. 2013). These associations between AHS, renal impairment, and allopurinol dose have led to the suggestion that excessive oxypurinol concentrations are a key causative factor. However, cases of AHS have been reported with concentrations within the proposed therapeutic range (30–100 µmol/L) (Casas et al. 1989; Emmerson et al. 1987; Puig et al. 1989), and many patients tolerate very high oxypurinol concentrations without adverse effects (Stamp et al. 2011a). Importantly, evidence suggests that sustained high oxypurinol concentrations after cessation of allopurinol in AHS patients with impaired renal function are associated with worse clinical outcomes (Chung et al. 2014). Excretion of oxypurinol may be increased with the use of uricosuric drugs, such as probenecid, or with haemodialysis (Elion et al. 1968). Given how rarely these severe adverse reactions occur, collaborative studies will be required to determine whether enhanced removal of oxypurinol by dialysis early in the course of AHS/SCAR improves outcomes. In the interim, early drug withdrawal and supportive care remain the mainstay of AHS management.

9.2 **Febuxostat**

Febuxostat is a potent non-purine inhibitor of both the oxidized and reduced forms of xanthine oxidase.

9.2.1 **Mechanism of action**

Febuxostat binds in a long, narrow channel leading to the molybdenum-pterin active site of xanthine oxidase, thereby preventing substrate binding and enzyme activity of the enzyme.

9.2.2 **Clinical pharmacology**

After oral administration, febuxostat is readily absorbed. It is metabolized in the liver by both conjugation via uridine diphosphate-glucuronosyltransferase (UGT) enzymes and oxidization to the active metabolites (67M-1, 67M-2, and 67M-4) by cytochrome P450 enzymes (CYP1A2, CYP2C8, and CYP2C9) (Grabowski et al. 2011; Mukoyoshi et al. 2008). The main route of elimination is via the kidneys, although some may be excreted in faeces. In patients with mild-moderate renal impairment, dose adjustment is not required. Studies of patients with more severe renal impairment are limited. In a study of 60 patients, of whom 67% had a eGFR <30 mL/min/1.72 m^2, low-dose febuxostat (mean 15.9 ± 8 mg daily) was associated with a significant reduction in serum urate and increase in eGFR (Sakai et al. 2014).

9.2.3 **Drug interactions**

Although it has not been formally tested, the combination of febuxostat and azathioprine should be avoided for the same reasons the allopurinol-azathioprine combination should be avoided. No significant interactions with a number of other medications frequently used in patients, including warfarin, colchicine, non-steroidal anti-inflammatories, and hydrochlorothiazide, have been reported.

9.2.4 **Clinical efficacy data**

Large clinical trials have established the efficacy of febuxostat in gout. Reduction in serum urate, tophus regression, and reduction in gout flares have all been reported. In the landmark studies of fixed-dose febuxostat, allopurinol has been the comparator urate-lowering therapy; the results are summarized in Table 9.2.

9.2.5 **Adverse effects**

Febuxostat is generally well tolerated. The most common adverse effects are diarrhoea, nausea, and abnormal liver function tests. Post-marketing cases of hepatic failure have been reported

Table 9.2 Results of key febuxostat vs allopurinol clinical trials		
Reference	**Study design**	**Results summary**
FACT study (n = 762) (Becker et al. 2005)	Patients with gout and SU ≥0.36 mmol/L randomized to febuxostat 80 mg/d, febuxostat 120 mg/d, or allopurinol 300 mg/d for 52 weeks	53% febuxostat 80 mg/d, 62% febuxostat 120 mg/d, and 21% allopurinol 300 mg/d achieved primary endpoint of SU <0.36 mmol/L at last 3 monthly visits Gout flares between weeks 9 and 52 occurred in 64% of patients on febuxostat 80 mg/d, 70% patients on febuxostat 120 mg/d, and 64% on allopurinol Median reduction in tophus area was 83% in febuxostat 80 mg/d, 66% in febuxostat 120 mg/d, and 50% in allopurinol
APEX study (n = 1072) (Schumacher et al. 2008)	Patients with gout and SU ≥0.48 mmol/L and creatinine ≤0.18 mmol/L randomized to febuxostat 80, 120, or 240 mg daily, or allopurinol 100 or 300 mg daily (depending on renal function) or placebo for 28 weeks	48% on febuxostat 80 mg/d, 65% on febuxostat 120 mg/d, 69% febuxostat on 240 mg/d, and 22% on allopurinol achieved primary endpoint of SU <0.36 mmol/L at last 3 monthly visits
CONFIRMS study (n = 2269) (Becker et al. 2010)	Patients with gout and SU ≥0.48 mmol/L and CrCL ≥30 mL/min randomized to febuxostat (40 or 80 mg/d), allopurinol (200 or 300 mg/d depending on renal function) for 28 weeks	In the group as a whole, 45% febuxostat 40 mg/d, 67% on febuxostat 80 mg/d, and 42% allopurinol achieved primary endpoint In subgroup with CrCL 30–89 mL/min, 50% febuxostat 40 mg/d, 72% on febuxostat 80 mg/d, and 42% allopurinol achieved primary endpoint of SU <0.36 mmol/L at the final visit
EXCEL study (n = 1086) (Becker et al. 2009)	3-year, open-label extension study febuxostat 80 or 120 mg/d vs allopurinol 300 mg/d	After one month SU<0.36 mmol/L in 81% febuxostat 80 mg/d, 87% febuxostat 120 mg/d, and 46% allopurinol Between 12 and 36 months 75–100% maintained target SU irrespective of treatment Maintenance of SU <0.36 mmol/L resulted in reduction in flare rates, with <4% patients having flares after 18 months of ULT irrespective of treatment arm Baseline tophus resolution achieved by 46% febuxostat 80 mg/d, 36% febuxostat 120 mg/d, and 29% allopurinol

(http://www.fda.gov/Safety/MedWatch/SafetyInformation/ucm243770.htm). Neutropaenia and rhabdomyolysis have been reported in patients with renal impairment (Kang et al. 2014; S. Kobayashi et al. 2013). Patients who have had allopurinol hypersensitivity may tolerate febuxostat, although caution is required, as some patients have developed rash or hypersensitivity with febuxostat (Abeles 2012).

9.3 **Probenecid**

Probenecid is a uricosuric agent that is typically, used in those patients who fail to achieve target serum urate with, cannot tolerate, or have contraindications to a xanthine oxidase inhibitor. It can be used as monotherapy or in combination with a xanthine oxidase inhibitor.

9.3.1 **Mechanism of action**

Probenecid inhibits the renal urate transporters URAT1 and GLUT9, resulting in normalization of renal urate excretion and a reduction in serum urate.

9.3.2 **Clinical pharmacology**

Probenecid is well absorbed after oral administration and has a half-life of 6–12 hours. Approximately 85–95% is bound to albumin. The main route of elimination is via the kidneys. As renal function declines so does the urate-lowering efficacy of probenecid (Bartels and Matossian 1959; Thompson et al. 1962). It has generally been considered to be a less effective urate-lowering therapy in patients with eGFR <50 mL/min/1.73 m^2, although this was not confirmed in a recent study (Pui et al. 2013).

9.3.3 **Drug interactions**

The interaction between probenecid and a number of antibiotics, including penicillin and β-lactam antibiotics, is specifically used to increase plasma antibiotic concentrations in some clinical situations. Aspirin, even in low dose, can reduce renal urate excretion (Caspi et al. 2000). However, aspirin does not appear have a clinically significant effect on the urate-lowering effects of probenecid (Harris et al. 2000). Probenecid reduces plasma oxypurinol in patients receiving concomitant allopurinol, although there does not appear to be an adverse effect on serum urate as a consequence (Stocker et al. 2008).

9.3.4 **Clinical efficacy data**

Probenecid is a moderately effectively urate-lowering therapy. In a small observational study, target serum urate was achieved in 33% of those receiving probenecid monotherapy and 37% of those receiving probenecid in combination with allopurinol (Pui et al. 2013). In another small study, patients failing to achieve target serum urate with allopurinol were randomized to receive either benzbromarone or probenecid. Ninety-two percent of patients who received benzbromarone achieved target serum urate compared to 65% who received probenecid ($p = 0.03$) (Reinders et al. 2009b). A recent Cochrane review concluded that benzbromarone is probably more successful than probenecid at achieving serum urate targets, and that benzbromarone resulted in fewer adverse events (Kydd et al. 2014).

9.3.5 **Adverse effects**

A significant proportion of patients report adverse effects associated with probenecid. In a study of 57 patients receiving probenecid, 18% reported adverse effects, most commonly gastrointestinal, and 12% of patients discontinued probenecid due to the adverse effects (Pui et al. 2013). Deposition of MSU crystals in the kidney and nephrolithiasis are other important adverse effects (Thompson et al. 1962).

9.4 **Benzbromarone**

Benzbromarone is a potent uricosuric. It is not widely available due to concerns over hepatotoxicity. However, it remains a useful therapeutic option, particularly in patients with significant renal impairment who have failed or have contraindications to xanthine oxidase and probenecid, and in transplant recipients who must remain on azathioprine.

9.4.1 **Mechanism of action**

Benzbromarone and one of its major metabolites, 6-hydroxybenzbromarone, act via the renal urate transporters URAT1 and GLUT9 to normalize renal uric acid excretion and thus lower serum urate.

9.4.2 **Clinical pharmacology**

Benzbromarone is primarily metabolized in the liver by CYP2C9 to 6-hydroxybenzbromarone and 1′-hydroxybenzbromarone (K. Kobayashi et al. 2012). The half-life of benzbromarone is ~3 hours, while that of 6-hydroxybenzbromarone is much longer. The majority of benzbromarone and its metabolites are excreted in bile and faeces, with a small amount (6%) excreted by the kidneys (Broekhuysen et al. 1972). Benzbromarone remains effective in patients with impaired renal function, although its ability to reduce serum urate declines as renal function declines, and when GFR is <20 mL/min, it may produce a reduction in serum urate of only ~20% (Heel et al. 1977; Masbernard and Giudicelli 1981).

9.4.3 **Drug interactions**

The important drug interactions are summarized in Table 9.1. Of particular relevance is the interaction between benzbromarone and warfarin, such that the anticoagulant effects of warfarin are increased. Consideration should be given to reducing the dose of warfarin by 30% and close monitoring of INR is required. Benzbromarone is hepatotoxic and caution is recommended when it is used in combination with other hepatotoxic drugs.

9.4.4 **Clinical efficacy data**

Benzbromarone is an effective urate-lowering therapy. In a small study of 65 patients, 26% of those receiving allopurinol 300 mg daily and 52% of those receiving benzbromarone 100 mg daily achieved serum urate <0.30 mmol/L (Reinders et al. 2009a). A greater percentage reduction in serum urate has been reported with benzbromarone compared to allopurinol (56.35% ± 10.98% vs. 32.81% ± 10.61%; p <0.001) (Perez-Ruiz et al. 1999). Benzbromarone has also been shown to reduce the size of tophi, alone and in combination with allopurinol (Perez-Ruiz et al. 2002).

9.4.5 **Adverse effects**

Benzbromarone is generally well tolerated, although gastrointestinal adverse effects, including diarrhoea, have been reported in 3.5% of patients receiving benzbromarone (Masbernard and Giudicelli 1981). The most feared adverse effect associated with benzbromarone is hepatotoxicity, which, although rare, can be fatal, especially with higher doses (e.g. 300 mg daily). For this reason a maximum dose of 100 mg daily is suggested. The risk of hepatotoxicity is increased with in those with pre-existing liver disease, a history of hepatotoxicity, and possibly excess alcohol intake. The risk of hepatotoxicity may be reduced by gradual dose increase and regular monitoring of liver function tests (Lee et al. 2008).

CYP2C9, which has a central role in the metabolism of benzbromarone, is subject to extensive genetic polymorphism. The poor metabolizer alleles *CYP2C9*2* (*rs1799853*, 430T>C, Arg144Cys) and *CYP2C9*3* (*rs1057910*, 1075A>C, Ile359Leu), which occur in 3–14% of Caucasians, 1–7% of Asians, and 3–5% of Polynesians, have been identified (Roberts et al. 2014; Scott et al. 2010). Genetic variations in *CYP2C9* have been shown to result in reduced clearance of benzbromarone (Uchida et al. 2010). Whether these genetic polymorphisms are associated with an increased risk of hepatotoxicity with benzbromarone remains to be determined.

9.5 **Pegloticase**

Recombinant uricases such as pegloticase are highly effective urate-lowering therapies, although due to their cost and requirement for intravenous administration, they are reserved for patients with severe refractory disease who have failed other conventional urate-lowering therapies.

Table 9.3 Dosing of urate-lowering therapies with renal or hepatic impairment

	Renal impairment	Hepatic impairment
Allopurinol	Starting dose: 50 mg/d if eGFR<60 mL/min and 100 mg/d if eGFR>60 mL/min Dosing in renal impairment controversial if fail to reach target SU on CrCL-based dose; gradual dose escalation while monitoring for adverse effects may be appropriate Haemodialysis: ~50% oxypurinol removed by dialysis, need to consider timing of dose in relation to dialysis	With current dosing guidelines no reduction required, but monitor LFT as increase above CrCL-based doses
Febuxostat	Mild-moderate: No dose adjustment required Severe: only small studies, lower doses used; remains effective at reducing SU Haemodialysis: limited data, but appears safe and effective (Sofue et al. 2014; Tojimbara et al. 2014)	Mild-moderate (Child Pugh class A or B); no dose adjustment required (Khosravan et al. 2006) Severe renal impairment; limited data; caution advised
Benzbromarone	Effective in patients with impaired renal function (GFR>20 mL/min) When GFR is <20 mL/min may produce a reduction in SU of only ~20%	Contraindicated due to risk of hepatotoxicity
Probenecid	Minimal data in renal impairment and no studies to determine the threshold CrCL below which probenecid would be expected to have a clinically insignificant urate-lowering effect Not recommended as first-line uricosuric in patients with CrCL<50 mL/min (Khanna et al. 2012)	No dose adjustment required
Pegloticase	Limited data in stage 3–4 chronic kidney disease remains effective and safe Haemodialysis: serum pegloticase concentrations unaffected, remained an effective urate-lowering therapy with no safety signal in one small study (Bleyer et al. 2015)	No dose adjustment required

9.5.1 **Mechanism of action**

Humans lack the enzyme uricase which metabolizes urate to allantoin, thus urate is the final product of purine metabolism (Figure 9.1). Pegloticase is a recombinant polyethylene glycol–conjugated uricase which thus metabolizes urate. Pegloticase is contraindicated in patients with glucose-6-phosphate dehydrogenase (G6PD) deficiency due to the risk of haemolysis and methemoglobinemia.

9.5.2 **Clinical pharmacology**

Pegloticase is administered by intravenous infusion every two weeks. Formation of anti-pegloticase antibodies occurs in ~40% and these antibodies are associated with a loss of urate-lowering effect (Lipsky et al. 2014). The risk of developing anti-drug antibodies may be reduced by concomitant use of immunosuppression (Hershfield et al. 2014). There is limited experience with pegloticase in patients with renal impairment. In a post-hoc analysis of two phase-3 pegloticase clinical trials which included patients with CKD stage 3 and 4, there was no significant change in renal function; the efficacy and safety of pegloticase did not appear to be affected by renal function (Yood et al. 2014).

9.5.3 **Drug interactions**

There are no specific drug interaction studies with pegloticase. Use with other biological agents is best avoided.

9.5.4 **Clinical efficacy data**

Pegloticase rapidly and profoundly reduces serum urate and can lead to resolution of gouty tophi (Baraf et al. 2013; Sundy et al. 2011). Because of the dramatic reduction in serum urate it can cause a significant number of gout flares in the short term despite the use of prophylactic therapy (Sundy et al. 2011).

9.5.5 **Adverse effects**

In the pegloticase clinical trials, infusion reactions were the most common adverse effect after gout flares, occurring in ~40% of patients. In a recent analysis of infusion reactions from the two clinical trials, they were generally mild to moderate, resolved with slowing or stopping the infusion, and were associated with a loss of pegloticase urate-lowering efficacy. Approximately 90% of all reactions occurred in those with a pre-infusion urate >0.36 mmol/L (Baraf et al. 2014). A recent analysis of the FDA adverse event reporting system found that cardiovascular events occurred more frequently than expected statistically (Gentry et al. 2014). Further data are required about the cardiovascular safety of pegloticase.

9.6 Summary

There are a number of effective urate-lowering therapies in the management of gout. The choice of agent is dictated by co-morbidities, particularly renal and hepatic impairment (summarized in Table 9.3).

References

Abeles AM (2012). Febuxostat hypersensitivity. *Journal of Rheumatology*, 39(3), 659.

Annemans L, et al. (2008). Gout in the UK and Germany: prevalence, comorbidities and management in general practice 2000–2005. *Annals of the Rheumatic Diseases*, 67(7), 960–66.

Baraf HS, et al. (2014). Infusion-related reactions with pegloticase, a recombinant uricase for the treatment of chronic gout refractory to conventional therapy. *Journal of Clinical Rheumatology*, 20(8), 427–32.

Baraf HS, et al. (2013). Tophus burden reduction with pegloticase: results from phase 3 randomized trials and open-label extension in patients with chronic gout refractory to conventional therapy. *Arthritis Research & Therapy*, 15(15), R137.

Bartels EC and Matossian GS (1959). Gout: six-year follow-up on probenecid therapy. *Arthritis & Rheumatism*, 2(3), 193–202.

Becker MA, et al. (2009). Clinical efficacy and safety of successful longterm urate lowering with febuxostat or allopurinol in subjects with gout. *Journal of Rheumatology*, 36, 1273–82.

Becker MA, et al. (2010). The urate-lowering efficacy and safety of febuxostat in the treatment of the hyperuricaemia of gout: the CONFIRMS trial. *Arthritis Research & Therapy*, 12, R63.

Becker MA, et al. (2005). Febuxostat compared with allopurinol in patients with hyperuricaemia and gout. *New England Journal of Medicine*, 353, 2450–61.

Bleyer AJ, Wright D, Alcorn H (2015). Pharmacokinetics and pharmacodynamics of pegloticase in patients with end-stage renal failure receiving hemodialysis. *Clinical Nephrology*, 83(5), 286–92.

Broekhuysen J, et al. (1972). Metabolism of benzbromarone in man. *European Journal of Clinical Pharmacology*, 4(2), 125–30.

Casas E, et al. (1989). The allopurinol hypersensitivity syndrome: its relation to plasma oxypurinol levels. *Advances in Experimental Medicine and Biology*, 253A, 257–60.

Caspi D, et al. (2000). The effect of mini-dose aspirin on renal function and uric acid handling in elderly patients. *Arthritis & Rheumatism*, 43(1), 103–08.

Chung W-H, et al. (2014). Insights into the poor prognosis of allopurinol-induced severe cutaneous adverse reactions: the impact of renal insufficiency, high plasma levels of oxypurinol and granulysin. *Annals of the Rheumatic Diseases*. doi:10.1136/annrheumdis-2014-205577

Dalbeth N, et al. (2006). Dose adjustment of allopurinol according to creatinine clearance does not provide adequate control of hyperuricaemia in patients with gout. *Journal of Rheumatology*, 33(8), 1646–50.

Day R, et al. (1988). Allopurinol dosage selection: relationships between dose and plasma oxypurinol and urate concentrations and urinary urate excretion. *British Journal of Clinical Pharmacology*, 26, 423–28.

Elion GB, et al. (1968). Renal clearance of oxipurinol, the chief metabolite of allopurinol. *American Journal of Medicine*, 45, 69–77.

Emmerson B, et al. (1987). Plasma oxypurinol concentrations during allopurinol therapy. *British Journal of Rheumatology*, 26, 445–49.

Gentry WM, et al. (2014). Investigation of pegloticase-associated adverse events from a nationwide reporting system database. *American Journal of Health-System Pharmacy*, 71(9), 722–7.

Grabowski BA, et al. (2011). Metabolism and excretion of [14C] febuxostat, a novel nonpurine selective inhibitor of xanthine oxidase, in healthy male subjects. *Journal of Clinical Pharmacology*, 51(2), 189–201.

Halevy S, et al. (2008). Allopurinol is the most common cause of Stevens-Johnson syndrome and toxic epidermal necrolysis in Europe and Israel. *Journal of the American Academy of Dermatology*, 58(1), 25–32.

Hande K, Noone R, Stone W (1984). Severe allopurinol toxicity: description and guidelines for prevention in patients with renal insufficiency. *American Journal of Medicine*, 76, 47–56.

Harris M, et al. (2000). Effect of low dose daily aspirin on serum urate levels and urinary excretion in patients receiving probenecid for gouty arthritis. *Journal of Rheumatology*, 27(12), 2873–6.

Harrold LR, et al. (2009). Adherence with urate-lowering therapies for the treatment of gout. *Arthritis Research & Therapy*, 11, R46.

Heel R, et al. (1977). Benzbromarone: A review of its pharmacological properties and therapeutic uses in gout and hyperuricaemia. *Drugs*, 14(5), 349–66.

Hershfield MS, et al. (2014). Induced and pre-existing anti-polyethylene glycol antibody in a trial of every 3-week dosing of pegloticase for refractory gout, including in organ transplant recipients. *Arthritis Research & Therapy*, 16, R63.

Hershfield MS, et al. (2013). Clinical Pharmacogenetics Implementation Consortium guidelines for human leukocyte antigen-B genotype and allopurinol dosing. *Clinical Pharmacology & Therapeutics*, 93(2), 153–8.

Jung JW, et al. (2015). An effective strategy to prevent allopurinol-induced hypersensitivity by HLA typing. *Genetics in Medicine*. doi:10.1038/gim.2014.195

Kang Y, et al. (2014). Rhabdomyolysis associated with initiation of febuxostat therapy for hyperuricaemia in a patient with chronic kidney disease. *Journal of Clinical Pharmacy and Therapeutics*, 39, 328–30.

Kardaun SH, et al. (2013). Drug reaction with eosinophilia and systemic symptoms (DRESS): an original multisystem adverse drug reaction. Results from the prospective RegiSCAR study. *British Journal of Dermatology*, 169, 1071–80.

Khanna D, et al. (2012). 2012 American College of Rheumatology Guidelines for the Management of Gout. Part 1: Systematic nonpharmacologic and pharmacologic therapeutic approaches to hyperuricaemia. *Arthritis Care & Research*, 64(10), 1431–46.

Khosravan R, et al. (2006). The effect of mild and moderate hepatic impairment on pharmacokinetics, pharmacodynamics, and safety of febuxostat, a novel nonpurine selective inhibitor of xanthine oxidase. *Journal of Clinical Pharmacology*, 46(1), 88–102.

Kobayashi K, et al. (2012). Identification of CYP isozymes involved in benzbromarone metabolism in human liver microsomes. *Biopharmaceutics & Drug Disposition*, 33, 466–73.

Kobayashi S, Ogura M, and Hosoya T (2013). Acute neutropenia associated with initiation of febuxostat therapy for hyperuricaemia in patients with chronic kidney disease. *Journal of Clinical Pharmacy and Therapeutics*, 38, 258–61.

Kydd ASR, et al. (2014). Uricosuric medications for chronic gout. *Cochrane Database of Systematic Reviews* 11, CD010457. doi: 10.1002/14651858.CD010457.pub2

Lee M-H, et al. (2008). A benefit-risk assessment of benzbromarone in the treatment of gout: was its withdrawal from the market in the best interests of patients? *Drug Safety*, 31(8), 643–65.

Lipsky PE, et al. (2014). Pegloticase immunogenicity: the relationship between efficacy and antibody development in patients treated for refractory chronic gout. *Arthritis Research & Therapy*, 16, R60.

Masbernard A and Giudicelli C (1981). Ten years' experience with benzbromarone in the management of gout and hyperuricaemia. *South African Medical Journal*, 59, 701–06.

McInnes G, Lawson D, Jick H (1981). Acute adverse reactions attributed to allopurinol in hospitalised patients. *Annals of the Rheumatic Diseases*, 40, 245–49.

Mukoyoshi M, et al. (2008). In vitro drug-drug interaction studies with febuxostat, a novel non-purine selective inhibitor of xanthine oxidase: plasma protein binding, identification of metabolic enzymes and cytochrome P450 inhibition. *Xenobiotica*, 38(5), 496–510.

Perez-Ruiz F, et al. (2002). Effect of urate-lowering therapy on the velocity of size reduction of tophi in chronic gout. *Arthritis Care & Research*, 47(4), 356–60.

Perez-Ruiz F, et al. (1999). Treatment of chronic gout in patients with renal function impairment: an open, randomised, actively controlled study. *Journal of Clinical Rheumatology* 5(2), 49–55.

Pui K, Gow PJ, Dalbeth N (2013). Efficacy and tolerability of probenecid as urate-lowering therapy in gout: clinical experience in high-prevalence population. *Journal of Rheumatology*, 40 (6), 872–6.

Puig J, et al. (1989). Plasma oxypurinol concentration in a patient with allopurinol hypersensitivity. *Journal of Rheumatology*, 16 (6), 842–44.

Ramasamy SN, et al. (2013). Allopurinol hypersensitivity: a systematic review of all published cases, 1950–2012. *Drug Safety*, 36, 953–80.

Reinders MK, et al. (2009a). A randomised controlled trial on the efficacy and tolerability with dose escalation of allopurinol 300–600mg/day versus benzbromarone 100–200 mg/day in patients with gout. *Annals of the Rheumatic Diseases*, 68, 892–97.

Reinders MK, et al. (2009b). Efficacy and tolerability of urate-lowering drugs in gout: a randomised controlled trial of benzbromarone versus probenecid after failure of allopurinol. *Annals of the Rheumatic Diseases*, 68, 51–56.

Riedel A, et al. (2004). Compliance with allopurinol therapy among managed care enrollees with gout: a retrospective analysis of administrative claims. *Journal of Rheumatology*, 31(8), 1575–81.

Roberts RL, et al. (2014). Frequency of CYP2C9 polymorphisms in Polynesian people and potential relevance to management of gout with benzbromarone. *Joint Bone Spine*, 81(2), 160–3.

Sakai Y, et al. (2014). Febuxostat for treating allopurinol-resistant hyperuricemia in patients with chronic kidney disease. *Renal Failure*, 36(2), 225–31.

Schumacher HR, et al. (2008). Effects of febuxostat versus allopurinol and placebo in reducing serum urate in subjects with hyperuricaemia and gout: a 28-week, phase III, randomized, double-blind, parallel-group trial. *Arthritis Care & Research*, 59(11), 1540–48.

Scott SA, et al. (2010). Combined CYP2C9, VKORC1 and CYP4F2 frequencies among racial and ethnic groups. *Pharmacogenomics*, 11, 781–91.

Sivera F, et al. (2014). Multinational evidence-based recommendations for the diagnosis and management of gout: integrating systematic literature review and expert opinion of a broad panel of rheumatologists in the 3e initiative. *Annals of the Rheumatic Diseases*, 73(2), 328–35.

Sofue T, et al. (2014). Efficacy and safety of febuxostat in the treatment of hyperuricemia in stable kidney transplant recipients. *Drug Design, Development and Therapy*, 8, 245–53.

Stamp LK, et al. (2006). Gout in renal transplant recipients. *Nephrology*, 11, 367–71.

Stamp LK, et al. (2011a). Relationship between serum urate and plasma oxypurinol in the management of gout: determination of minimum plasma oxypurinol concentration to achieve a target serum urate level. *Clinical Pharmacology & Therapeutics*, 90(3), 392–8.

Stamp LK, et al. (2011b). Using allopurinol above the dose based on creatinine clearance is effective and safe in chronic gout, including in those with renal impairment. *Arthritis & Rheumatism*, 63(2), 412–21.

Stamp LK, et al. (2012a). Furosemide increases plasma oxypurinol without lowering serum urate – a complex drug interaction: implications for clinical practice. *Rheumatology*, 51(9), 1670–6.

Stamp LK, et al. (2012b). Starting dose, but not maximum maintenance dose, is a risk factor for allopurinol hypersensitivity syndrome: a proposed safe starting dose of allopurinol. *Arthritis & Rheumatism*, 64(8), 2529–36.

Stocker SL, et al. (2008). Pharmacokinetic and pharmacodynamic interaction between allopurinol and probenecid in healthy subjects. *Clinical Pharmacokinetics*, 47(2), 111–18.

Sundy JS, et al. (2011). Efficacy and tolerability of pegloticase for the treatment of chronic gout in patients refractory to conventional treatment: two randomized controlled trials. *Journal of the American Medical Association*, 306(7), 711–20.

Thompson GR, et al. (1962). Long term uricosuric therapy in gouty. *Arthritis & Rheumatism*, 5, 384–96.

Tojimbara T, et al. (2014). Efficacy and safety of febuxostat, a novel nonpurine selective inhibitor of xanthine oxidase for the treatment of hyperuricemia in kidney transplant recipients. *Transplantation Proceedings*, 46, 511–13.

Uchida S, et al. (2010). Benzbromarone pharmacokinetics and pharmacodynamics in different cytochrome P450 2C9 genotypes. *Drug Metabolism and Pharmacokinetics* 25, 605–10.

Venkat Raman G, Sharman V, Lee H (1990). Azathioprine and allopurinol: a potentially dangerous combination. *Journal of Internal Medicine*, 228, 69–71.

Yood RA, et al. (2014). Effect of pegloticase on renal function in patients with chronic kidney disease: a post hoc subgroup analysis of 2 randomized, placebo-controlled, phase 3 clinical trials. *BMC Research Notes*, 7, 54.

Chapter 10

Anti-inflammatory agents for prophylaxis and flares

> **Key points**
> - Acute gout requires rapid, effective treatment.
> - Colchicine, non-steroidal anti-inflammatories, and corticosteroids are all effective; the choice of agent is dictated by the patient's co-morbidities and concomitant medications.
> - Interleukin-1 inhibitors are effective, but the high cost precludes routine use, and long-term safety data for repeated use are lacking.

The goal of acute gout management is rapid, effective suppression of the inflammatory response. Colchicine, non-steroidal anti-inflammatories, and corticosteroids are the mainstay of acute gout management and have been available for many years. Interleukin (IL)-1 inhibitors are a new addition to the therapeutic armamentarium for acute gout. These same agents can be used in patients commencing urate-lowering therapy as prophylaxis against acute gout flare. The choice of agent is dictated by the patient's co-morbidities and concomitant medications. Each of the therapeutic options will be discussed in detail in this chapter.

10.1 Colchicine

Colchicine, an alkaloid extracted from saffron or crocus, has been used in the treatment of gout since the time of Hippocrates. It has a narrow therapeutic index and there is a high mortality associated with overdose (Jayaprakash et al. 2007). This has led to increased awareness of appropriate dosing regimens, especially in the elderly and those with renal impairment. Despite the concerns, there is evidence for efficacy in acute gout and for low-dose prophylaxis in patients commencing urate-lowering therapy.

10.1.1 Mechanism of action

The majority of the anti-inflammatory effects of colchicine are a result of its binding to tubulin, thus preventing the formation of microtubulin heterodimers which are involved in cell division, signal transduction, regulation of gene expression, and migration (Terkeltaub 2009). Colchicine has also been shown to supress monosodium urate (MSU)–induced NALP3 inflammasome activity in macrophages (Martinon et al. 2006). Activated neutrophils recruited to inflamed joints are an important line of defence against MSU crystals. Colchicine has a number of effects on neutrophils, including alteration in adhesion molecule expression, thereby reducing neutrophil adhesion and recruitment into inflamed joints (Cronstein et al. 1995) and inhibition of a specific and characteristic protein tyrosine phosphorylation pattern that is induced when neutrophils are exposed to MSU crystals (Roberge et al. 1993). Other anti-inflammatory effects of colchicine are reviewed extensively elsewhere (Nuki 2008; Terkeltaub 2009).

10.1.2 **Clinical pharmacology**

Colchicine is readily absorbed after oral ingestion in the jejenum and ileum. Oral bioavailability is ~45%. Colchicine is primarily eliminated via enterohepatic recirculation and biliary excretion, with 10–20% eliminated via the kidneys. Dose reduction is therefore recommended in patients with hepatic and/or renal impairment (see Section 10.1.6 on dosing).

10.1.3 **Drug interactions**

Important interactions between colchicine and cytochrome P45 3A4 (CYP3A4) and P-glycoprotein (Gp) inhibitors have been identified. CYP3A4 has a role in the metabolism of colchicine to its inactive metabolites, while P-Gp is thought to limit gastrointestinal absorption of colchicine. Co-administration of colchicine and CYP3A4 or P-Gp inhibitors can therefore result in accumulation of colchicine and toxicity. For example, verapamil, a CYP3A4 and P-Gp inhibitor, decreases colchicine clearance by ~50% and thus increases plasma colchicine concentrations (Terkeltaub et al. 2009).

10.1.4 **Clinical efficacy data**

10.1.4.1 **Acute gout**

Surprisingly, there are only two placebo-controlled trials of colchicine in the management of acute gout. A small study in 43 patients undertaken in the late 1980s compared placebo and colchicine 1 mg stat followed by 0.5 mg every two hours until complete response or toxicity (e.g. nausea, vomiting, and diarrhoea). Although colchicine was more effective in reducing pain, it was associated with significant gastrointestinal adverse effects which usually occurred before clinical benefit (Ahern et al. 1987). The Acute Gout Flare Receiving Colchicine Evaluation (AGREE) trial randomized 184 patients to either low-dose colchicine (1.2 mg stat then 0.6 mg at one hour), high-dose colchicine (1.2 mg stat then 0.6 mg hourly for 6 hours), or placebo. Both high- and low-dose colchicine were significantly more effective than placebo. There was no significant difference between the two colchicine regimens on pain reduction, but the higher dose strategy was associated with significantly more adverse effects (Terkeltaub et al. 2010).

10.1.4.2 **Prophylaxis**

Colchicine has been shown to be effective as prophylaxis against acute gout in patients commencing urate-lowering therapy. In a 6-month study of 43 patients commencing allopurinol, colchicine 0.6 mg bd was associated with significantly fewer flares compared to placebo (0.52 vs. 2.91; $p = 0.008$) (Borstad et al. 2004). In patients commencing probenecid, similar results were observed (Paulus et al. 1974).

10.1.5 **Adverse effects**

The most common adverse effects of colchicine are gastrointestinal, including nausea and diarrhoea. In general these gastrointestinal adverse effects are dose dependent (Terkeltaub et al. 2010). Other less common adverse effects include bone marrow suppression and neuromyotoxicity (Kuncl et al. 1987). Impaired kidney function (CrCL<50 ml/min) is reported to be a predictor of these less common adverse effects (Wallace et al. 1991). Because of the risk, it has been suggested that a full blood count and creatine kinase should be checked every 6 months in patients with CrCL<50 ml/min who are receiving long-term prophylactic oral colchicine, defined as 0.5 mg daily for ≥6 months (Mikuls et al. 2004).

10.1.6 **Dosing**

The recommended colchicine dosing in acute gout has reduced since the publication of the AGREE trial, with the current FDA-approved dose at 1.2 mg stat followed by 0.6 mg one hour later. Further dose reduction may be required in elderly patients and those with renal impairment. For prophylaxis against gout when commencing urate-lowering therapy, a dose of 0.6 mg once or twice daily is generally sufficient.

10.2 **NSAIDs and COX-2 inhibitors**

There are six main classes of non-steroidal anti-inflammatory drugs (NSAIDs); at least 20 different NSAIDs are available. There is variability in dose, duration of action, and efficacy, with some patients responding better to one NSAID than others. In general, NSAIDs should be used at the lowest dose possible for the shortest period of time to reduce the risk of adverse effects.

10.2.1 **Mechanism of action**

The key mechanism of action of NSAIDs is inhibition of cyclo-oxygenase (COX), resulting in decreased conversion of arachidonic acid to the pro-inflammatory prostaglandins, prostacyclin and thromboxanes. There are two isoforms of COX, namely COX-1 and COX-2. Most traditional NSAIDs inhibit both isoforms, while the newer COX-2 inhibitors are relatively selective in their inhibition of COX-2.

10.2.2 **Clinical pharmacology**

There are a large number of NSAIDs available. These can be classified according to chemical structure into several groups (Table 10.1). In general, NSAIDs are well absorbed. There is variability in half-life: as shown in Table 10.1, the can be divided into short- (<6 hours) or long- (>6 hours) acting. NSAIDs are generally metabolized by the liver and excreted by the kidneys.

10.2.3 **Drug interactions**

NSAIDs have multiple drug interactions, which may be of particular importance to gout patients with co-morbidities. NSAIDs may interact with anti-coagulants to increase the risk of bleeding and may antagonize the blood pressure lowering effects of antihypertensive agents. Concomitant use of a NSAID and corticosteroids may increase the risk of gastrointestinal adverse effects. Particularly concerning is the use of an NSAID, an angiotensin-converting enzyme (ACE) inhibitor, and a diuretic in combination, which may have adverse effects on blood pressure and renal function.

Table 10.1 NSAID groupings (not exhaustive)

Group	Available NSAID	Long- or short-acting
Propionic acids	Naproxen Ibuprofen Ketoprofen	Long Short Short
Acetic acids	Diclofenac Indometacin Sulindac	Short Short Long
Oxicams (enolic acids)	Meloxicam Piroxicam	Long Long
Salicylates	Aspirin (acetylated) Diflunisal (non-acetylated)	Long
Selective COX-2	Celecoxib	Long

10.2.4 **Clinical efficacy data**

10.2.4.1 *Acute gout*

The efficacy of NSAIDs and some newer COX-2 inhibitors in the management of acute gout has been demonstrated in a number of clinical trials (Alloway et al. 1993; Altman et al. 1988; Janssens et al. 2008; Man et al. 2007; Rubin et al. 2004; Schumacher et al. 2002, 2010). There is no current evidence to suggest any one NSAID is superior to another; the choice of specific NSAID or COX-2 inhibitor will depend on the patient's co-morbidities and response to NSAIDs in the past. Early institution of NSAID at the highest-tolerated or maximum dose is the key to success in treating acute gout. While NSAIDs may be an appropriate first-line treatment for younger patients with gout, there are many patients with gout who are elderly, have co-morbidities, or concomitant medications that preclude the use of NSAIDs for the management of gout.

10.2.4.2 *Prophylaxis*

There are surprisingly little data on the use of NSAIDs as prophylaxis when commencing urate-lowering therapy (ULT). One study examined the effects of azapropazone with allopurinol and reported a benefit with respect to gout attacks but with an increased rate of adverse effects (Daymond et al. 1983).

10.2.5 **Adverse effects**

The adverse effects with NSAIDs are well recognized. Gastrointestinal adverse effects include ulceration, bleeding, and perforation. NSAIDs may have multiple adverse effects on the kidney, including acute renal failure due to renal vasoconstriction, hypertension, and electrolyte disturbance, including hyperkalaemia. In individuals with pre-existing renal or cardiac disease, NSAIDs may lead to a worsening of renal function. Mild increases in hepatic transaminases are also common. NSAIDs have also been associated with an increased risk of major cardiovascular events, such as myocardial infarction, stroke, and death. In a recent meta-analysis of >300,000 participants from >600 trials after 1 year, there was a significantly increased risk of major cardiovascular events with diclofenac and the coxibs but not with naproxen (Bhala et al. 2013).

10.3 **Corticosteroids**

Oral, intravenous (IV), intra-muscular (IM), and intra-articular (IA) corticosteroids can all be used in the management of acute gout. IA corticosteroid may be particularly useful when only one or two large joints are involved. Acute gout and septic arthritis may be difficult to distinguish clinically and may co-exist, so care must be taken to exclude septic arthritis before administration of IA corticosteroid.

10.3.1 **Mechanism of action**

Corticosteroids exert their effects by binding to the glucocorticoid receptor and glucocorticoid response elements on genomic DNA, thereby regulating transcription of a large number of target genes. There are a wide range of anti-inflammatory effects of corticosteroids, including decreased neutrophil adhesion and inhibition of pro-inflammatory cytokines, including IL-1β, IL-6, IL-17, and TNF, which are involved in gouty arthritis.

10.3.2 **Clinical pharmacology**

Orally administered corticosteroids such as prednisone and prednisolone are well absorbed and have high oral bioavailability. Corticosteroids, with the exception of prednisolone, are two-thirds weakly bound to albumin with one-third freely circulating. Only the unbound fraction is pharmacologically active. Corticosteroids are metabolized in the liver to inactive metabolites which are excreted by the kidneys.

10.3.3 **Drug interactions**

Corticosteroids are metabolized by CYP3A4; thus medications that strongly induce or inhibit CYP3A4 may alter corticosteroid concentrations. Of particular relevance in gout, there is no evidence for an interaction between corticosteroids and ULTs.

10.3.4 **Clinical efficacy data**

10.3.4.1 *Acute gout*

Oral, IV, IM, and IA steroid have all been used in the management of acute gout. Oral prednisolone 35 mg daily for 5 days has been shown to be as effective as naproxen 500 mg BD for 5 days in the management of gout as determined by reduction in pain scores at 90 hours (reduction 44.7 mm vs. 46.0 mm, respectively) (Janssens et al. 2008). Similarly, the combination of oral prednisolone 30 mg daily for 5 days in combination with prn paracetamol was as effective as IM diclofenac 75 mg followed by indometacin 50 mg tds for 2 days and 25 mg tds for 3 days in combination with prn paracetamol with respect to pain relief.

Not surprisingly, there were fewer adverse effects associated with oral prednisolone (Man et al. 2007). The prednisolone strategy was also more cost-effective, at least in part due to the occurrence of gastrointestinal haemorrhage requiring hospital admission in six patients receiving indometacin (Cattermole et al. 2009). In a small study of 27 patients presenting within 5 days of crystal-proven gout, IM triamcinolone 60 mg was as safe and effective as indometacin 50 mg tid for at least 2 days. Complete resolution of symptoms occurred after an average of 8 days in the indometacin group and 7 days in the triamcinolone group (Alloway et al. 1993). IA corticosteroids, although accepted as an effective treatment, have not been well studied. One small uncontrolled trial reported improvement of symptoms within 48 hours with IA injection of triamcinolone acetonide 10 mg in knees and 8 mg in small joints (Fernandez et al. 1999).

10.3.4.2 *Prophylaxis*

Given the adverse effects associated with long-term corticosteroid use, their use should be reserved for those patients where colchicine and NSAIDs are contraindicated, poorly tolerated, or ineffective. The risks and benefits of corticosteroid for prophylaxis should be considered for each individual patient; the dose of prednisone should be $\leq$10 mg daily (Khanna et al. 2012).

10.3.5 **Adverse effects**

Corticosteroids, particularly when given at high doses or over a prolonged period, are associated with a wide range of adverse effects (Table 10.2). Of particular relevance in the management of gout are the adverse effects of IA corticosteroid, which include pain, fat necrosis, and iatrogenic infection. The risk of iatrogenic infection is difficult to ascertain accurately, but appears to be low, with reports ranging from 1:13,900 to 1:77,300 (Gray and Gottlieb 1983; Seror et al. 1999).

10.3.6 **Dosing**

The dose of corticosteroid depends on the drug, route of administration, and size of the joint. In general, oral prednisone 30–40 mg daily for 1–2 days followed by a slow taper over 1–2 weeks is used in the management of gout. More rapid tapering of prednisone can be associated with a rebound flare.

Table 10.2 Common adverse effects associated with corticosteroids	
Gastrointestinal	Gastritis Peptic ulcer Steatohepatitis Pancreatitis
Bone	Osteoporosis Avascular necrosis
Central nervous system	Insomnia Anxiety Mood alterations
Dermatologic	Hirsutism Skin thinning Acne Bruising
Endocrine	Diabetes Pituitary-adrenal axis suppression Sodium and water retention
Ocular	Cataracts Glaucoma
Neuromuscular	Muscle atrophy and weakness

10.4 **IL-1 inhibitors**

IL-1 is a key pro-inflammatory cytokine involved in acute gout and as such is a potential therapeutic target (see Chapter 2). There are currently three IL-1 inhibitors available: rilonacept, anakinra, and canakinumab. Of these, canakinumab has been most studied in the management of acute gout and prophylaxis during initiation of ULT. The use of these drugs in acute gout is the subject of ongoing clinical investigation. Currently no IL-1 inhibitors are FDA-approved for acute gout; only canakinumab is approved by the EMA for use in acute gout.

10.4.1 **Mechanism of action**

Rilonacept is a fully human recombinant soluble decoy receptor protein that binds IL-1α and IL-1β, thereby preventing binding to and activation of cell surface receptors. Canakinumab is a fully human anti-IL-1β monoclonal antibody. Anakinra is a recombinant IL-1 receptor antagonist (IL-1Ra) that binds IL-1R, thereby preventing IL-1α and IL-1β receptor binding.

10.4.2 **Drug interactions**

There are no formal studies examining drug interactions with IL-1 inhibitors. In general, IL-1 inhibitors should not be used in combination with other biologic agents such as TNF inhibitors due to the increased risk of infections and neutropaenia.

High levels of IL-1 supresses the formation of CYP450, an important enzyme in drug metabolism. Thus IL-1 inhibition could lead to normalization of CYP450 formation. A number of drugs are metabolized by CYP450, leading to the potential for drug interactions. This might be most important for drugs with a narrow therapeutic index, such as warfarin or anti-convulsants; appropriate monitoring should be undertaken.

10.4.3 **Clinical efficacy data**

10.4.3.1 *Acute gout*

In patients unresponsive or with contraindications to NSAIDs and colchicine, subcutaneous canakinumab has been reported to have a significantly greater and more rapid reduction in pain, joint tenderness, and swelling compared to IM triamcinolone in the treatment of acute gout (Schlesinger et al. 2011a, 2012; So et al. 2010). Other markers of inflammation, such as CRP and serum amyloid A, are also significantly reduced in those who received canakinumab compared to triamcinolone (Schlesinger et al. 2011a, 2012). Importantly, health-related quality of life as measured by SF 36 and the gout impact scale are significantly improved with canakinumab as compared to IM triamcinolone (Hirsch et al. 2014; Schlesinger et al. 2011a). Interestingly, a single dose of canakinumab also reduces the risk of recurrent flares over 8 weeks (relative risk reduction 94%, canakinumab 150 mg vs. triamcinolone acetonide 40 mg) (So et al. 2010).

There is one study of rilonacept in the treatment of acute gout. In this phase-three, randomized, double-blind, double-dummy active and placebo-controlled study, 225 patients were randomized to treatment with SC placebo plus oral indometacin 50 mg tds for 3 days, then 25 mg tds for up to 9 days; SC rilonacept 320 mg plus oral placebo tds for 3 days, then tds for up to 9 days; or SC rilonacept 320 mg plus oral indometacin 50 mg tds for 3 days, then 25 mg tds for up to 9 days. Although there was a greater reduction in pain in the rilonacept-plus-indometacin vs. indometacin-alone groups, this did not reach statistical significance (-1.55 ± 0.92 vs. -1.40 ± 0.96; $p = 0.33$) (Terkeltaub et al. 2013).

The effects of anakinra in acute gout are limited to retrospective case series and one small uncontrolled of pilot study of ten patients (Ghosh et al. 2013; Ottaviani et al. 2013; So et al. 2007). In all these reports, anakinara was well tolerated and resulted in improvements, signs, and symptoms of acute gout. Further large clinical trials are required.

10.4.3.2 *Prophylaxis*

The effects of canakinumab on the risk of gout flares in patients commencing allopurinol for the treatment of gout has been examined in one study. Patients ($n = 432$) were randomized to canakinumab 25, 50, 100, 200, or 300 mg SC; 4 × 4 weekly doses of canakinumab; or oral colchicine 0.5 mg daily for 16 weeks. Significantly fewer patients experienced ≥1 gout flare with all canakinumab doses compared to colchicine: 15–27% vs. 44%; $p < 0.05$). At canakinumab doses ≥50 mg, there was a 64–72% reduction in the risk of ≥1 gout flare at 16 weeks compared to colchicine (Schlesinger et al. 2011b).

Rilonacept has also been shown to reduce the frequency of gout flares during the initiation of ULT in two phase-three, randomized, placebo-controlled studies (Mitha et al. 2013; Schumacher et al. 2012). In the larger study, 248 patients commencing allopurinol were randomized to once-weekly SC placebo, rilonacept 80 mg, or rilonacept 160 mg for 16 weeks. The proportion of patients with no flares during the study period was significantly higher in the rilonacept groups compared to placebo (rilonacept 80 mg: 74.4%, rilonacept 160 mg: 79.5%, placebo: 43.9%; $p \leq 0.0001$) (Mitha et al. 2013).

10.4.4 **Adverse effects**

Injection-site reactions and infections are the most common adverse effects associated with rilonacept and canakinumab. Infections were reported in 20%, serious infections in 1.8%, and injection-site reactions in 4.9% of the 225 patients receiving canakinumab in the 12-week β-RELIEVED and β-RELIEVED II studies (Schlesinger et al. 2012). Although an increase in thrombocytopenia, neutropenia, and low white blood cells was noted in the canakinumab

Table 10.3 Important drug interactions with medications used to treat acute gout

	Drugs which may interact	Effect	Dosing adjustment	Monitoring required
NSAIDs	Warfarin	Increased risk GI bleeding		INR
	ACE inhibitors	Hypertension and potential for deterioration in renal function		Creatinine Blood pressure
Colchicine	CYP3A4 and p-glycoprotein inhibitors (e.g. diltiazem, verapamil, ciclosporin, clarithromycin)	Increased risk of colchicine-induced toxic effects	Reduce colchicine dose by 33–66%	FBC, CK
Corticosteroids	Warfarin	Increased risk GI bleeding		
	CYP3A4	Corticosteroids metabolized by CYP3A4		

group compared to those who received the comparator agent triamcinolone, these abnormalities were not associated with an increased risk of clinical infections or bleeding.

In the majority of canakinumab studies, patients have received a single dose of drug. In the β-RELIEVED and β-RELIEVED II studies (Schlesinger et al. 2012), a small number of patients (n = 60) received re-treatment, and in another study, 54 patients received canakinumab 4 weekly × 4 (Schlesinger et al. 2011b), with no increase in adverse events or serious adverse events observed. However, further long-term safety data, particularly in patients who require repeated doses of an IL-1 inhibitor, are required.

10.5 **Combination therapy**

Combination therapy is common in the management of acute gout (Gnanenthiran et al. 2011; Schlesinger et al. 2006). The most frequently used combinations are NSAID and IA corticosteroid, NSAID and oral corticosteroid, and NSAIDs and colchicine. Combination therapy is reserved for those patients with severe acute gout and those with acute polyarticular gout. Recommended combinations include colchicine with NSAIDs or oral corticosteroids, or IA steroid with NSAID, colchicine or oral steroid (Khanna et al. 2012).

10.6 **Summary and international guidelines**

Each of the therapies available for the management of acute gout have beneficial effects and unique potential adverse effects. The choice of agent is generally dictated by the patient's co-morbidities and concomitant medications, with consideration to important drug interactions (summarized in Table 10.3). Currently available international guidelines on the use of these agents are outlined in Table 10.4.

Table 10.4 Comparison of international recommendations for acute gout treatment

Drug for acute gout	ACR 2012 guidelines (Khanna et al. 2012)	EULAR 2006 guidelines (Zhang et al. 2006)	BSR 2007 guidelines (Jordan et al. 2007)
• **Colchicine**	• Appropriate first-line if attack onset <36 hours and no contraindications • Loading dose of 1.2 mg followed by 0.6 mg 1 hour later which can be followed by gout attack prophylaxis dosing 0.6 mg once or twice daily 12 hours later, until the gout attack resolves • If only 1.0 mg or 0.5 mg tablets of colchicine are available, loading dose of 1.0 mg colchicine followed by 0.5 mg 1 hour later, and then followed, as needed, after 12 hours, by continued colchicine (up to 0.5 mg 3 times daily) until the acute attack resolves	• Appropriate as first-line therapy if no contraindications • 0.5 mg three times daily	• Colchicine can be an effective alternative to NSAID but is slower to work • Doses of 0.5 mg bd–qds in order to diminish the risks of adverse effects
• **NSAIDs**	• Acceptable first-line treatment at full dose	• NSAID convenient and well-accepted option: first-line	• Fast-acting NSAIDs in maximum doses drug of choice
• **Steroids**	• Oral, IM, or IA can be used as first-line depending on the number and size of joint involved	• IA steroid safe and effective – useful if NSAID or colchicine contraindicated	• IA steroids effective • Oral, IA, IM, or IV if fail to tolerate NSAIDs or refractory to other treatments
• **IL-1 inhibitors**	• Not considered	• Not considered	• Not considered

References

Ahern M, et al. (1987). Does Colchicine really work? the results of the first controlled study in acute gout. *Australian and New Zealand Journal of Medicine*, 17, 301–04.

Alloway J, et al. (1993). Comparison of triamcinolone acetonide with indomethacin in the treatment of acute gouty arthritis. *Journal of Rheumatology*, 20(1), 111–13.

Altman RD, et al. (1988). Ketoprofen versus indomethacin in patients with acute gouty arthritis: a multicenter, double blind comparative study. *Journal of Rheumatology*, 15(9), 1422–26.

Bhala N, et al. (2013). Vascular and upper gastrointestinal effects of non-steroidal anti-inflammatory drugs: meta-analyses of individual participant data from randomised trials. *Lancet*, 382(9894), 769–79.

Borstad GC, et al. (2004). Colchicine for prophylaxis of acute flares when initiating allopurinol for chronic gouty arthritis. *Journal of Rheumatology*, 31, 2429–32.

Cattermole GN, et al. (2009). Oral prednisolone is more cost-effective than oral indomethacin for treating patients with acute gout-like arthritis. *European Journal of Emergency Medicine*, 16, 261–66.

Cronstein BN, et al. (1995). Colchicine alters the quantitative and qualitative display of selectins on endothelial cells and neutrophils. *Journal of Clinical Investigation*, 96, 994–1002.

Daymond TJ, Laws D, Templeton JS (1983). A comparison of azapropazone and allopurinol in the treatment of chronic gout. *British Journal of Clinical Pharmacology*, 15, 157.

Fernandez C, et al. (1999). Treatment of acute attacks of gout with a small dose of intraarticular triamcinolone acetonide. *Journal of Rheumatology*, 26(10), 2285–86.

Ghosh P, et al. (2013). Treatment of acute gouty arthritis in complex hospitalized patients with anakinra. *Arthritis Care & Research*, 65(8), 1381–84.

Gnanenthiran SR, et al. (2011). Acute gout management during hospitalization: a need for a protocol. *Internal Medicine Journal*, 41(8), 610–7.

Gray RG and Gottlieb NL (1983). Intra-articular corticosteroids: an updated assessment. *Clinical Orthopaedics and Related Research*, 177, 235–63.

Hirsch JD, et al. (2014). Efficacy of Canakinumab vs. triamacinolone acetonide according to multiple gouty arthritis-related health outcome measures. *International Journal of Clinical Practice*, 68(12), 1503–7.

Janssens HJ, et al. (2008). Use of oral prednisolone or naproxen for the treatment of gout arthritis: a double-blind, randomised equivalence trial. *Lancet*, 371, 1854–60.

Jayaprakash V, Ansell G, Galler D (2007). Colchicine overdose: the devil is in the detail. *New Zealand Medical Journal*, 120(1248).

Jordan KM, et al. (2007). British Society for Rheumatology and British Health Professionals in Rheumatology guideline for the management of gout. *Rheumatology*, 46(8), 1372–74.

Khanna D, et al. (2012). 2012 American College of Rheumatology Guidelines for the Management of Gout. Part 2: Therapy and antiinflammatory prophylaxis of acute gouty arthritis. *Arthritis Care & Research*, 64(10), 1447–61.

Kuncl R, et al. (1987). Colchicine myopathy and neuropathy. *New England Journal of Medicine*, 316(25), 1562–68.

Man CY, et al. (2007). Comparison of oral prednisolone/paracetamol and oral indomethacin/paracetamol combination therapy in the treatment of acute gout like arthritis: a double-blind, randomized, controlled trial. *Annals of Emergency Medicine*, 49(5), 670–77.

Martinon F, et al. (2006). Gout-associated uric acid crystals activate the NALP3 inflammasome. *Nature*, 440, 237–41.

Mikuls T, et al. (2004). Quality of care indicators for gout management. *Arthritis & Rheumatism*, 50(3), 937–43.

Mitha E, et al. (2013). Rilonacept for acute gout flare during initiation of uric acid lowering therapy: results from the PRESURGE-2 international, phase 3, randomized, placebo-controlled trial. *Rheumatology*, 52, 1285–92.

Nuki G (2008). Colchicine: its mechanism of action and efficacy in crystal-induced inflammation. *Current Rheumatology Reports*, 10, 218–77.

Ottaviani S, et al. (2013). Efficacy of anakinra in gouty arthritis: a retrospective study of 40 cases. *Arthritis Research & Therapy*, 15, R123.

Paulus HE, et al. (1974). Prophylactic colchicine therapy of intercritical gout: a placebo-controlled study of probenecid-treated patients. *Arthritis & Rheumatism*, 17(5), 609–14.

Roberge CJ, et al. (1993). Crystal-induced neutrophil activation. IV. Specific inhibition of tyrosine phosphorylation by colchicine. *Journal of Clinical Investigation*, 92, 1722–29.

Rubin B, et al. (2004). Efficacy and safety profile of treatment with etoricoxib 120 mg once daily compared with indomethacin 50 mg three times daily in acute gout. *Arthritis & Rheumatism*, 50(2), 598–606.

Schlesinger N, et al. (2006). A survey of current evaluation and treatment of gout. *Journal of Rheumatology*, 33(10), 2050–52.

Schlesinger N, et al. (2011a). Canakinumab relieves symptoms of acute flares and improves health-related quality of life in patients with difficult to treat gouty arthritis by suppressing inflammation: results of a randomised, dose-ranging study. *Arthritis Research & Therapy*, 13, R53.

Schlesinger N, et al. (2011b). Canakinumab reduces the risk of acute gouty arthritis flares during initiation of allopurinol treatment: results of a double-blind, randomised study. *Annals of the Rheumatic Diseases*, 70, 1264–71.

Schlesinger N, et al. (2012). Canakinumab for acute gouty arthritis in patients with limited treatment options: results from two randomised, multicentre, active-controlled, double blind trials and their initial extensions. *Annals of the Rheumatic Diseases*, 71, 1839–48.

Schumacher HR, et al. (2010). Efficacy and tolerability of celecoxib in the treatment of moderate to extreme pain associated with acute gouty arthritis: a randomized controlled trial. *Arthritis & Rheumatism*, 62(10 [(Suppl)), S63.

Schumacher HR, et al. (2002). Randomised double blind trial of etoricoxib and indomethacin in treatment of acute gouty arthritis. *BMJ*, 324, 1488–92.

Schumacher HR, et al. (2012). Rilonacept (interleukin-1 trap) for prevention of gout flares during initiation of uric acid–lowering therapy: results from a phase III randomized, double-blind, placebo-controlled, confirmatory efficacy study. *Arthritis Care & Research*, 64(10), 1462–70.

Seror P, et al. (1999). Frequency of sepsis after local corticosteroid injection (an inquiry on 1160000 injections in rheumatological private practice in France). *Rheumatology*, 38 (12), 1272–4.

So A, et al. (2007). A pilot study of IL-1 inhibition by anakinra in acute gout. *Arthritis Research & Therapy*, 9, R28.

So A, et al. (2010). Canakinumab for the treatment of acute flares in difficult-to-treat gouty arthritis. Results of a multicenter, phase II, dose ranging study. *Arthritis & Rheumatism*, 62(10), 3064–76.

Terkeltaub R (2009). Colchicine update: 2008. *Seminars in Arthritis & Rheumatism*, 38(6), 411–9.

Terkeltaub R, et al. (2009). New dosing guidelines for colchicine to avoid toxicity when used with Ca2+ channel blockers: the potent P-Gp/CYP3A4 inhibitor verapamil increases maximal concentration of single dose colchicine by 30% and exposure by ~100% in healthy subjects. *Arthritis & Rheumatism*, 60(10 [Suppl]), S414.

Terkeltaub R, et al. (2010). High versus low dosing of oral colchicine for early acute gout flare. *Arthritis & Rheumatism*, 62(4), 1060–68.

Terkeltaub R, et al. (2013). Rilonacept in the treatment of acute gouty arthritis: a randomized, controlled clinical trial using indomethacin as the active comparator. *Arthritis Research & Therapy*, 15, R25.

Wallace S, et al. (1991). Renal function predicts colchicine toxicity: guidelines for the prophylactic use of colchicine in gout. *Journal of Rheumatology*, 18(2), 264–69.

Zhang W, et al. (2006). EULAR evidence based recommendations for gout. Part II: Management. Report of a task force of the EULAR Standing Committee for International Clinical Studies Including Therapeutics (ESCISIT). *Annals of the Rheumatic Diseases*, 65(10), 1312–24.

Chapter 11

Management of co-morbid conditions in people with gout

Key points

- Co-morbidities—particularly hypertension, cardiovascular disease, renal impairment, diabetes, obesity, and hyperlipidaemia—are common in gout.
- Patients with gout should be screened for co-morbidities.
- Co-morbidities will influence choice of therapy for acute gout flares and urate lowering.

Gout is associated with a number of co-morbidities, including hypertension, cardiovascular disease, renal impairment, diabetes, obesity, and hyperlipidaemia. These co-morbidities frequently occur in combination and are collectively known as the metabolic syndrome. The presence of co-morbidities and medications used in their management may have an effect on the development of gout as well as implications for the management of gout. This chapter will discuss the interaction between key co-morbidities and gout, and recommendations for screening for co-morbidities.

11.1 Hypertension

Hyperuricaemia/gout and hypertension frequently co-exist. In the 2007–2008 National Health and Nutrition Examination Survey (NHANES), hypertension was present in 74% of patients with gout and 47% of those with hyperuricaemia (defined as serum urate >7.0 mg/dL in men and >5.7 mg/dL in women) but no history of gout (Zhu et al. 2012). Urate may have a causal role in hypertension (Feig et al. 2008; Mazzali et al. 2010).

A number of medications used in the management of hypertension influence serum urate (Table 11.1). For example, loop and thiazide diuretics increase serum urate, while amlodipine, a calcium channel blocker, and losartan, an angiotensin II receptor antagonist, reduce serum urate (Burnier et al. 1993; Chanard et al. 2003; Sennesael et al. 1996). In patients with difficulty achieving target serum urate, controlling gout, or both, consideration should be given to the most appropriate antihypertensive agent. This is particularly important with those receiving furosemide, which not only increases serum urate but also attenuates the hypouricaemic effects of allopurinol and oxypurinol in patients with gout (Stamp et al. 2012).

Urate-lowering therapies may also have effects on blood pressure. Allopurinol has been reported to reduce blood pressure in hyperuricaemic adults and adolescents with essential hypertension (Feig et al. 2010; Kanbay et al. 2007). While there are no specific studies on the effects of febuxostat on blood pressure, a significant reduction in blood pressure was observed in a study of hyperuricaemic patients undergoing cardiac surgery who were treated with up to 60 mg daily of febuxostat for 6 months (Sezai et al. 2013). One small study in pre-hypertensive, obese adolescents randomized patients to allopurinol 100 mg bd for 1

Table 11.1 Effect of cardiovascular medications on serum urate concentrations

	Increase serum urate	No effect on serum urate	Lower serum urate	Reference
Antihypertensives		Lisinopril	Losartan ACE inhibitors (captopril, enalapril, ramipril) Calcium channel blockers (e.g. amlodipine, felodipine)	Burnier et al. 1993; Soffer et al. 1995 Chanard et al. 2003; Sennesael et al. 1996
	Beta blockers (propranolol, atenolol, metoprolol, timolol, alprenolol)			Reyes 2003
Diuretics	Furosemide Thiazides	Spironolactone		Garcia Puig et al. 1991; Tiitinen et al. 1983
Lipid-lowering agents		Simvastatin	Atorvastatin Fenofibrate	Milionis et al. 2004 Desager et al. 1980; Feher et al. 2003; Takahashi et al. 2003
Aspirin	Low doses (60–300 mg/d) reduce renal urate excretion, may increase serum urate	Doses >1 g/d increase renal urate excretion and lower serum urate		Caspi et al. 2000

Source: Stamp and Chapman (2012).

week then 200 mg bd for 7 weeks, probenecid 250 mg daily for a week then 500 mg bd for 7 weeks, or placebo. At the end of the 8-week study, those receiving allopurinol or probenecid had a significant reduction in serum urate and in blood pressure as compared to placebo. However, there was no difference between allopurinol and probenecid with respect to urate or blood pressure reduction (Soletsky and Feig 2012). These data suggest that the blood pressure lowering effects are related to a reduction in urate rather than inhibition of xanthine oxidase. There is currently insufficient evidence to suggest that urate-lowering therapies should be used routinely in the management of hypertension in the absence of gout (Gois and Souza 2013).

11.2 **Cardiovascular disease**

Hyperuricaemia has been associated with an increased risk of cardiovascular disease, although a causal relationship has not been established (Feig et al. 2008; SY Kim et al. 2010). Recent Mendelian randomization studies have reported conflicting results: one suggested high urate is causally related to adverse cardiovascular outcomes, particularly sudden cardiac death (Kleber et al. 2015); the other reported no association (Palmer et al. 2013).

Gout has been associated with an increased risk of coronary artery disease (Choi and Curhan 2007; De Vera et al. 2010; Krishnan et al. 2006; Zhu et al. 2012), death due to cardiovascular causes (Stack et al. 2013; Teng et al. 2012), stroke (Seminog and Goldacre 2013), peripheral artery disease (Baker et al. 2007), and heart failure (Krishnan 2013). The risk of cardiovascular disease in patients with gout also appears to differ between men and women, with a stronger association observed in women (Clarson et al. 2015; De Vera et al. 2010). Medications such as aspirin and beta blockers, which are frequently used in the management of cardiovascular disease, may also increase serum urate (Table 11.1).

The effects of urate-lowering therapy on cardiovascular outcomes in patients with and without gout is the subject of ongoing investigation. In a large, retrospective, nested case-controlled study of 25,090 patients with heart failure, a history of gout as well as a recent acute episode of gout (≤60 days), allopurinol use was associated with a significant reduction in heart failure readmissions or death (RR = 0.69; 95% CI [0.60, 0.79]) and reduced all-cause mortality (RR = 0.74; 95% CI [0.61, 0.90]) (Thansaaoulis et al. 2010). In hyperuricaemic patients with heart failure, urate lowering with benzbromarone had no effect on cardiac haemodynamics despite reducing serum urate (Ogino et al. 2010). These results suggest that inhibition of xanthine oxidase rather that urate lowering per se may be important.

Several recent studies have examined the effects of allopurinol on cardiovascular outcomes. In a case-controlled study of 2277 patients with their first myocardial infarct and 4849 matched controls, allopurinol use was reported in 3.1% and 3.8%, respectively. Allopurinol use was associated with a 20% reduction in risk of myocardial infarction (Grimaldi-Bensouda et al. 2015). There were too few patients with gout in this study receiving alternate urate-lowering therapy or no urate-lowering therapy to examine the effects of allopurinol in the subgroup with gout.

In another retrospective cohort study of Taiwanese patients with gout and no prior history of cardiovascular disease, those receiving allopurinol (n = 2483) were matched on a 1:1 ratio by age, gender, diabetes, hypertension, and hyperlipidaemia with those not receiving allopurinol. Patients were not matched on presence of chronic kidney disease, and there were significantly more patients in the allopurinol group with chronic kidney disease. Important cardiovascular risk factors such as blood pressure and smoking were also not available in the cohort. Importantly, 69% of patients in the non-allopurinol group were receiving a uricosuric agent, most commonly benzbromarone. This study concluded that allopurinol appeared to increase the risk—and uricosuric therapy to reduce the risk—of cardiovascular events (Kok et al. 2014). However, the majority of patients in this study were receiving ≤100 mg daily of allopurinol, with only 15% receiving ≥300 mg daily. Those patients receiving higher doses of allopurinol had a lower risk of cardiovascular events compared to those on low dose, suggesting that the dose of allopurinol and the degree of serum urate reduction may be important (Kok et al. 2014).

Another cohort study compared gout patients commencing a xanthine oxidase inhibitor with no urate-lowering therapy. It observed neither an increased nor a decreased cardiovascular risk (SC Kim et al. 2015b).

Well-designed, prospective clinical trials are now required to determine the effects of urate-lowering therapy on cardiovascular outcomes, and to determine whether a specific target urate needs to be achieved to observe clinical benefit. One phase-3b randomized trial is currently underway in 7500 gout patients with well-defined cardiovascular disease. The aim is to compare the risk of major adverse cardiovascular events (cardiovascular death, nonfatal myocardial infarction, nonfatal stroke, and unstable angina with urgent revascularization) in patients on febuxostat and allopurinol (White et al. 2012). Unfortunately, there are no placebo or uricosuric arms in this study.

Some studies suggest that colchicine may have a role in secondary prevention of cardiovascular disease. In a prospective, randomized controlled trial of patients with stable coronary artery disease, the addition of colchicine 0.5 mg daily to standard secondary prevention strategies was associated with a reduction in the combined outcomes of acute coronary syndrome, out-of-hospital cardiac arrest, and non-cardioembolic ischaemic stroke (HR = 0.33; 95% CI [0.18, 0.59]; p <0.001) (Nidorf et al. 2013). Colchicine may be an appropriate choice for those patients with cardiovascular disease where NSAIDs are contraindicated, although potential drug interactions must be considered (see Chapter 10).

11.3 Renal impairment

There are well-recognized, complex relationships between hyperuricaemia, gout, and renal function. Creatinine is one of the most important determinants of serum urate; creatinine clearance, which is a better indicator of renal function as it adjusts for some of the variability in creatinine due to age, weight, and gender, correlates inversely with serum urate.

Hyperuricaemia (serum urate > 0.41 mmol/L) is an independent risk factor for the development and progression of renal impairment (Bellomo et al. 2010; Ficociello et al. 2010; Ohno et al. 2001). Chronic kidney disease is also a risk factor for development of gout (W. Wang et al. 2015b). Gout is common in patients with chronic kidney disease: ~70% patients with gout are reported to have an estimated glomerular filtration rate (eGFR) < 60 mL/min per 1.73 m^2; 20% have an eGFR < 30 mL/min per 1.73 m^2 (Zhu et al. 2012).

Clinicians managing gout need to be mindful of how therapies for gout may influence or be influenced by chronic kidney disease. NSAIDs and colchicine are contraindicated in patients with renal impairment. Allopurinol dosing remains controversial in chronic kidney disease; it is discussed in detail in Chapter 9. Effective urate lowering in patients with gout improves renal function, although at least part of this may relate to reduced NSAID use in those with adequately controlled gout (Perez-Ruiz et al. 2000). A post-hoc analysis of the FOCUS study demonstrated that urate lowering with febuxostat in patients with gout was associated with an improvement in renal function (Whelton et al. 2011).

The effect of urate-lowering therapy on progression of kidney disease is the subject of ongoing investigation. A meta-analysis, which included eight studies of allopurinol in a total of 476 participants, reported no significant difference in the change in eGFR from baseline between allopurinol and control group in five of the studies (mean difference = 3.1 mL/min/1.73 m^2, 95% CI [−0.9, 7.1]; p = 0.1). In three studies, allopurinol was associated with a small decrease in creatinine from baseline (mean difference = −0.4 mg/dL, 95% CI [−0.8, –0.0]; p = 0.03) (Bose et al. 2014). Another study reported that in hyperuricaemic patients with chronic kidney disease, stage-3 febuxostat for 12 weeks had no effect on creatinine or GFR (Tanaka et al. 2015). Currently there is insufficient evidence to recommend use of allopurinol or febuxostat to slow the progression of chronic kidney disease. Randomized, placebo-controlled trials are currently underway which will provide further evidence of the risks and benefits of urate-lowering therapy in patients with chronic kidney disease.

11.4 Diabetes

A case-controlled, nested study from a UK General Practice database reported a reduced risk of incident gout in patients with diabetes (RR = 0.67; 95% CI [0.63, 0.71]) compared to patients without diabetes (Rodriguez et al. 2010). This inverse relationship was stronger for patients with type 1 diabetes than those with type 2 diabetes. This reduced risk of incident gout in patients with diabetes may relate to the uricosuric effect of glycosuria (Cook et al. 1986) and the impaired inflammatory responses observed in diabetes.

Conversely, it appears there is an increased risk of incident diabetes in patients with gout. In a large study using data from a USA insurance plan, the risk of incident diabetes was increased in patients with gout compared to osteoarthritis after adjusting for a number of confounding variables, including age, co-morbidities, and medications (incidence rate = 1.71; 95% CI [1.62, 1.81]) (SC Kim et al. 2015a). Furthermore, the risk of incident diabetes was higher in women than men. Similar findings of increased risk of incident diabetes in patients with gout compared to non-gout, and in women compared to men, have been reported using data from the UK Health Improvement network (Rho et al. 2014).

Whether management of gout with urate-lowering therapy reduces the risk of future diabetes is unknown. One retrospective study examined the association between colchicine use and risk of diabetes in patients with gout. There was a trend towards decreased risk of diabetes in those who had received colchicine, although this did not reach statistical significance (L. Wang et al. 2015a).

11.5 Obesity

Over 50% of patients with gout are reported to be obese (Zhu et al. 2012), and a high BMI predisposes individuals to gout (Campion et al. 1987; Lee et al. 2015). Obesity is one of the strongest modifiable risk factors associated with gout.

Weight loss in obese individuals results in a reduction in serum urate (Heyden 1978; Nicholls and Scott 1972). In a small study of 13 patients with gout, weight loss was associated with a reduction in serum urate (baseline serum urate = 9.6 ± 1.7 mg/dL, falling to 7.9 ± 1.5 mg/dL; $p = 0.001$), along with a decrease in frequency of gouty attacks (from 2.1 ± 0.8 attacks/month to 0.6 ± 0.7 attacks/month; $p = 0.002$) (Dessein et al. 2000). Bariatric surgery, which usually leads to substantial weight loss, has also been associated with a significant reduction in serum urate and gout attacks (Dalbeth et al. 2014; Romero-Talamás et al. 2014).

11.6 Combinations of co-morbidities

The interaction between urate, co-morbidities, and gout are complex, with some co-morbidities being both cause and effect of hyperuricaemia. Hypertension, cardiovascular disease, renal impairment, diabetes, obesity, and hyperlipidaemia frequently occur in combination and are collectively known as the *metabolic syndrome*. Using NHANES 1988–1994 data, the prevalence of metabolic syndrome was 62.8% (95% CI [51.9, 73.6]) among those with gout and 25.4% (95% CI [23.5, 27.3]) among those without gout (Choi and Ford 2007).

It has been suggested that there may be other different combinations of these important co-morbidities in gout. In a cross-sectional study of 2763 patients with gout cluster, analysis revealed five different patterns of co-morbidities associated with gout (Table 11.2) (Richette et al. 2015). The authors suggest that these clinical phenotypes may reflect different pathophysiological processes linked to gout.

11.7 Screening for co-morbid conditions in people with gout

Current guidelines recommend screening patients with gout for associated co-morbidities, including obesity, diabetes, hypertension, hyperlipidaemia, and modifiable risk factors for cardiovascular disease (Khanna et al. 2012; Zhang et al. 2006) (Table 11.3). Given the high prevalence of co-morbidities in patients with gout, the ease of screening for them, and given that appropriate management of these co-morbidities may have a beneficial effect on long-term health, screening should be encouraged despite the lack of causal association between gout and

Table 11.2 Frequency of co-morbidities in patients with gout

Cluster	Hypertension (≥130/85 mmHg or current treatment)	Diabetes (fasting glucose >1.26 g/L or current treatment)	Obesity (BMI >30 kg/m^2)	Dyslipidaemia	Cardiovascular disease (history of angina and/or MI)	Renal impairment eGFR <60 mL/min	MS
1 n = 332 (12%)	145 (44%)	0 (0)	0 (0)	0 (0)	0 (0)	0 (0)	48 (34%)
2 n = 483 (17%)	308 (64%)	0 (0)	483 (100%)	362 (75%)	0 (0)	0 (0)	226 (66%)
3 n = 664 (24%)	513 (77%)	499 (75%)	371 (56%)	541 (81%)	16 (2%)	9 (1%)	391 (77%)
4 n = 782 (28%)	447 (57%)	17 (2%)	15 (2%)	770 (98%)	6 (1%)	2 (0)	307 (48%)
5 n = 502 (18%)	466 (93%)	167 (33%)	196 (39%)	391 (78%)	252 (50%)	230 (46%)	258 (68%)

Source: Richette et al. (2015)

Table 11.3 Summary of associations between co-morbidities and hyperuricaemia/gout

Co-morbidity	Evidence for association in observational studies	Evidence for association in Mendelian randomization studies	Effect of urate-lowering therapy on co-morbidity
Hypertension	Hyperuricaemia associated with increased risk of incident hypertension RR 1.4; 95% CI [1.23, 1.58] (Grayson et al. 2011)	No evidence of causal association between urate and hypertension (Palmer et al. 2013)	Allopurinol, febuxostat, and probenecid shown to reduce blood pressure in small studies Insufficient evidence to recommend urate-lowering therapy for hypertension in the absence of gout
Cardiovascular disease	Hyperuricaemia associated with increased risk of CHD incidence (RR = 1.09; 95% CI [1.03, 1.16] and for CHD mortality (RR = 1.16, 95% CI [1.01, 1.30] (SY Kim et al. 2010) Gout has been associated with an increased risk of coronary artery disease (Choi and Curhan 2007; De Vera et al. 2010; Krishnan et al. 2006; Zhu et al. 2012), death due to cardiovascular causes (Stack et al. 2013; Teng et al. 2012), stroke (Seminog and Goldacre 2013), peripheral artery disease (Baker et al. 2007), and heart failure (Krishnan 2013)	No evidence of causal association between urate and cardiovascular disease (Palmer et al. 2013) Evidence of causal association between urate and adverse cardiovascular outcomes, particularly sudden cardiac death (Kleber et al. 2015)	Data on urate-lowering therapy conflicting Ongoing clinical trials on the effects of urate-lowering therapy on cardiovascular disease in those with and without gout Currently insufficient evidence to recommend urate-lowering therapy for cardiovascular disease in the absence of gout
Renal impairment	Serum urate >0.40 mmol/L) is an independent risk factor for the development and progression of renal impairment (Bellomo et al. 2010; Ficociello et al. 2010; Ohno et al. 2001) Chronic kidney disease is associated with gout; among men, HR = 1.88, 95% CI [1.13, 3.13] among women, HR = 2.31, 95% CI [1.25, 4.24] (W. Wang et al. 2015b)	One study suggests activity of renal urate transporters in increasing serum urate is beneficial to renal function (Hughes et al. 2013)	Conflicting evidence on the effect of urate-lowering therapy on renal function in patients without gout (Bose et al. 2014) In patients with gout, urate lowering improves renal function Insufficient evidence to recommend urate-lowering therapy in patients with chronic kidney disease in the absence of gout Clinical trials ongoing
Diabetes	Increased risk of incident diabetes in patients with gout (SC Kim et al. 2015a; Rho et al. 2014)	No evidence	No evidence
Obesity	BMI associated with increased risk of gout (Campion et al. 1987; Lee et al. 2015)	No evidence	No evidence

some co-morbidities. Primary care physicians will have a key role in undertaking co-morbidity screening given that the majority of gout patients are managed in primary care. Appropriate systems need to be developed to ensure gout patients receive the recommended screening and management of co-morbidities.

References

Baker JF, Schumacher HR, and Krishnan E (2007). Serum uric acid level and risk for peripheral arterial disease: analysis of data from the multiple risk factor intervention trial. *Angiology*, 58(4), 450–7.

Bellomo G, et al. (2010). Association of uric acid with change in kidney function in healthy normotensive individuals. *American Journal of Kidney Diseases*, 56, 264–73.

Bose B, et al. (2014). Effects of uric acid-lowering therapy on renal outcomes: a systematic review and meta-analysis. *Nephrology Dialysis Transplantation*, 29, 406–13.

Burnier M, et al. (1993). Salt-dependent renal effects of an angiotensin II antagonist in healthy subjects. *Hypertension*, 22, 339–47.

Campion EW, Glynn R, and DeLabry LO (1987). Asymptomatic hyperuricaemia: risks and consequence in the normative aging study. *American Journal of Medicine*, 82, 421–26.

Caspi D, et al. (2000). The effect of mini-dose aspirin on renal function and uric acid handling in elderly patients. *Arthritis & Rheumatism*, 43(1), 103–08.

Chanard J, et al. (2003). Amlodipine reduces cyclosporin-induced hyperuricaemia in hypertensive renal transplant recipients. *Nephrology Dialysis Transplantation*, 18, 2147–53.

Choi HK and Curhan G (2007). Independent impact of gout on mortality and risk for coronary heart disease. *Circulation*, 116, 894–900.

Choi HK and Ford E (2007). Prevalence of the metabolic syndrome in individuals with hyperuricemia. *American Journal of Medicine*, 120, 442–7.

Clarson LE, et al. (2015). Increased risk of vascular disease associated with gout: a retrospective, matched cohort study in the UK Clinical Practice Research Datalink. *Annals of the Rheumatic Diseases*, 74, 642–47.

Cook DG, et al. (1986). Serum uric acid, serum glucose and diabetes: relationships in a population study. *Postgraduate Medical Journal*, 62, 1001–06.

Dalbeth N, et al. (2014). Impact of bariatric surgery on serum urate targets in people with morbid obesity and diabetes: a prospective longitudinal study. *Annals of the Rheumatic Diseases*, 73, 797–802.

De Vera MA, et al. (2010). The independent impact of gout on the risk of acute myocardial infarction among elderly women: a population-based study. *Annals of the Rheumatic Diseases*, 69(6), 1162–64.

Desager JP, Hulhoven R, and Harvengt C (1980). Uricosuric effect of fenofibrate in healthy volunteers. *Journal of Clinical Pharmacology*, 20, 560–64.

Dessein P, et al. (2000). Beneficial effects of weight loss associated with moderate calorie/carbohydrate restriction, and increased proportional intake of protein and unsaturated fat on serum urate and lipoprotein levels in gout: a pilot study. *Annals of the Rheumatic Diseases*, 59, 539–43.

Feher M, et al. (2003). Fenofibrate enhances urate reduction in men treated with allopurinol for hyperuricaemia and gout. *Rheumatology*, 42(2), 321–25.

Feig DI, Kang H-R, and Johnson RJ (2008). Uric acid and cardiovascular risk. *New England Journal of Medicine*, 359, 1811–21.

Feig DI, Soletsky B, and Johnson RJ (2010). Effect of allopurinol on blood pressure of adolescents with newly diagnosed essential hypertension. *Journal of the American Medical Association*, 300(8), 924–32.

Ficociello LH, et al. (2010). High-normal serum uric acid increases risk of early progressive renal function loss in type 1 diabetes. *Diabetes Care*, 33(6), 1337–43.

Garcia Puig J, et al. (1991). Hydrochlorathiazide vs. spironolactone: long term metabolic complications in patients with essential hypertension. *Journal of Clinical Pharmacology*, 31(5), 455–61.

Gois PHF and Souza ERDM (2013). Pharmacotherapy for hyperuricemia in hypertensive patients. *Cochrane Database of Systematic Reviews* 1, CD008652. doi: 10.1002/14651858.CD008652.pub2

Grayson PC, et al. (2011). Hyperuricemia and incident hypertension: a systematic review and meta-analysis. *Arthritis Care & Research*, 63(1), 102–10.

Grimaldi-Bensouda L, et al. (2015). Impact of allopurinol on the risk of myocardial infarction. *Annals of the Rheumatic Diseases*, 74, 836–42.

Heyden S (1978). The workingman's diet. II Effect of weight reduction in obese patients with hypertension, diabetes, hyperuricemia and hyperlipidemia. *Ann Nutr Metab*, 22(3), 141–59.

Hughes K, et al. (2013). Mendelian randomization analysis associates increased serum urate, due to genetic variation in uric acid transporters, with improved renal function. *Kidney Internationol*, 85(2), 344–51.

Kanbay M, et al. (2007). Effect of treatment of hyperuricemia with allopurinol on blood pressure, creatinine clearance, and proteinuria in patients with normal renal function. *International Urology and Nephrology*, 39(4), 1227–33.

Khanna D, et al. (2012), 2012 American College of Rheumatology Guidelines for the Management of Gout. Part 1: Systematic nonpharmacologic and pharmacologic therapeutic approaches to hyperuricaemia. *Arthritis Care & Research*, 64(10), 1431–46.

Kim SC, Liu J, and Solomon DH (2015a). Risk of incident diabetes in patients with gout: a cohort study. *Arthritis & Rheumatism*, 67(1), 273–80.

Kim SC, et al. (2015b). Effects of xanthine oxidase inhibition on cardiovascular disease in patients with gout: A cohort study. *American Journal of Medicine*, 128(6), 653.e7–53.

Kim SY, et al. (2010). Hyperuricaemia and coronary heart disease: a systematic review and meta-analysis. *Arthritis Care & Research*, 62(2), 170–80.

Kleber ME, et al. (2015). Uric acid and cardiovascular events. *Journal of the American Society of Nephrology*, doi: ASN0201407660

Kok VC, et al. (2014). Allopurinol therapy in gout patients does not associate with beneficial cardiovascular outcomes: a population based matched-cohort study. *PLoS One*, 9(6), e99102.

Krishnan E (2013). Gout and the risk for incident heart failure and systolic dysfunction. *BMJ Open*, 15(2), e000282.

Krishnan E, et al. (2006). Gout and the risk of acute myocardial infarction. *Arthritis & Rheumatism*, 54(8), 2688–96.

Lee J, et al. (2015). Visceral fat obesity is highly associated with primary gout in a metabolically obese but normal weighted population: a case control study. Arthritis Research & Therapy, 17(79).

Mazzali M, et al. (2010). Uric acid and hypertension: cause or effect? Current Rheumatology Reports, 12, 108–17.

Milionis H, et al. (2004). Effects of statin treatment on uric acid homeostasis in patients with primary hyperlipidaemia. American Heart Journal, 148, 635–40.

Nicholls A and Scott JT (1972). Effect of weight loss on plasma and urinary levels of uric acid. Lancet, 300, 1223–24.

Nidorf SM, et al. (2013). Low-dose colchicine for secondary prevention of cardiovascular disease. Journal of the American College of Cardiology, 61(4), 404–10.

Ogino K, et al. (2010). Uric acid lowering treatment with benzbromarone in patients with heart failure: a double-blind placebo-controlled cross-over preliminary study. Circulation: Heart Failure, 3(1), 73–81.

Ohno I, et al. (2001). Serum uric acid and renal prognosis in patients with IgA nephropathy. Nephron, 87(4), 333–39.

Palmer TM, et al. (2013). Association of plasma uric acid with ischaemic heart disease and blood pressure: mendelian randomisation analysis of two large cohorts. BMJ, 347(f4262). doi: 10.1136/bmj.f4262

Perez-Ruiz F, et al. (2000). Improvement of renal function in patients with chronic gout after proper control of hyperuricaemia and gouty bouts. Nephron, 86, 287–91.

Reyes A (2003). Cardiovascular drugs and serum uric acid. Cardiovascular Drugs and Therapy, 17(5/6), 397–414.

Rho YH, et al. (2014). Independent impact of gout on the risk of diabetes among women and men: a population based BMI-matched cohort study', Annals of the Rheumatic Diseases. doi:10.1136/annrheumdis-2014-205827

Richette P, et al. (2015). Revisiting co-morbidities in gout: a cluster analysis. Annals of the Rheumatic Diseases, 74, 142–7.

Rodriguez G, Soriano LC, and Choi HK (2010). Impact of diabetes against the future risk of developing gout. Annals of the Rheumatic Diseases, 69, 2090–94.

Romero-Talamás H, et al. (2014). The effect of bariatric surgery on gout: a comparative study. Surgery for Obesity and Related Diseases, 10, 1161–65.

Seminog OO and Goldacre MJ (2013). Gout as a risk factor for myocardial infarction and stroke in England: evidence from record linkage studies. Rheumatology, 52, 2251–59.

Sennesael J, et al. (1996). Divergent effects of calcium channel and angiotensin converting enzyme blockade on glomerulotubular function in cyclosporin-treated renal allograft recipients. American Journal of Kidney Diseases, 27(5), 701–08.

Sezai A, et al. (2013). Comparison of febuxostat and allopurinol for hyperuricemia in cardiac surgery patients (NU-FLASH Trial). Circulation Journal, 77, 2043–49.

Soffer B, et al. (1995). Effects of losartan on a background of hydrochlorothiazide in patients with hypertension. Hypertension, 26(1), 112–17.

Soletsky B and Feig DI (2012). Uric acid reduction rectifies prehypertension in obese adolescents. Hypertension, 60, 1148–56.

Stack AG, et al. (2013). Independent and conjoint associations of gout and hyperuricaemia with total and cardiovascular mortality. QJM, 106(4), 647–58.

Stamp LK and Chapman PT (2012). Gout and its co-morbidities: Implications for therapy. Rheumatology, 52(1), 34–44.

Stamp LK, et al. (2012). Furosemide increases plasma oxypurinol without lowering serum urate—a complex drug interaction: implications for clinical practice. Rheumatology, 51(9), 1670–6.

Takahashi S, et al. (2003). Effects of combination treatment using anti-hyperuricaemic agents with fenofibrate and/or losartan on uric acid metabolism. Annals of the Rheumatic Diseases, 62, 572–75.

Tanaka K, et al. (2015). Renoprotective effects of febuxostat in hyperuricemic patients with chronic kidney disease: a parallel-group, randomized, controlled trial. Clinical and Experimental Nephrology. doi: 10.1007/s10157-015-1095-1

Teng GG, et al. (2012). Mortality due to coronary heart disease and kidney disease among middle-aged and elderly men and women with gout in the Singapore Chinese Health Study. Annals of the Rheumatic Diseases, 71, 924–28.

Thansaaoulis G, et al. (2010). Gout, allopurinol use and heart failure outcomes. Archives of Internal Medicine, 170(15), 1358–64.

Tiitinen S, et al. (1983). Effect of nonsteroidal anti-inflammatory drugs on the renal excretion of uric acid. Clinical Rheumatology, 2(3), 233–36.

Wang L, et al. (2015a). Association between colchicine and risk of diabetes among the veterans affairs population with gout. Clinical Therapeutics. doi: 10.1016/j.clinthera.2015.03.010

Wang W, Bhole V, and Krishnan E (2015b). Chronic kidney disease as a risk factor for incident gout among men and women: retrospective cohort study using data from the Framingham Heart Study. BMJ Open, 5, e006843.

Whelton A, et al. (2011). Renal function in gout: long-term treatment effects of febuxostat. Journal of Clinical Rheumatology, 17(1), 7–13.

White WB, et al. (2012). Cardiovascular safety of febuxostat and allopurinol in patients with gout and cardiovascular comorbidities. American Heart Journal, 164(1), 14–20.

Zhang W, et al. (2006). EULAR evidence based recommendations for gout. Part II: Management. report of a task force of the EULAR Standing Committee for International Clinical Studies Including Therapeutics (ESCISIT). Annals of the Rheumatic Diseases, 65(10), 1312–24.

Zhu Y, Pandya BJ, and Choi HK (2012). Comorbidities of gout and hyperuricemia in the us general population: NHANES 2007–2008. American Journal of Medicine, 125, 679–87.

Chapter 12

Gout research tools: a summary for clinicians

Key points
• Although most tools used in gout research are generic, there are some important gout-specific instruments. • New gout classification criteria were published in 2015. • Outcome measure domains have been identified for both acute and chronic gout studies. • A preliminary flare definition has been reported. • Gout-specific, patient-reported outcome measure instruments allow assessment of gout disease activity and impact of tophi. • Imaging scoring systems allow quantification of joint damage, inflammation, and urate burden in gout.

Many of the outcome measure domains and tools used in gout research are generic and widely used in clinical studies of other rheumatic diseases. However, gout research has particular methodological challenges due to the fluctuating nature and the varied manifestations of the disease. There has been major progress in the definition and standardization of research tools for use in gout clinical studies. Understanding these concepts is essential for gout researchers but also important for clinicians when assessing the medical literature to guide clinical decision making for patients with gout. In this chapter, we describe the key tools that are used in gout clinical research.

12.1 Classification criteria

Classification criteria are used to ensure relative homogeneity of participants in clinical research, including clinical trials and epidemiological studies. A number of gout classification criteria have been described. Until recently the most frequently used criteria were the 1977 American Rheumatism Association preliminary criteria for the classification of the acute arthritis of primary gout (Wallace et al. 1977). However, clinical criteria not requiring synovial fluid analysis have low sensitivity and specificity (<80%) in both early and established disease, with particularly low specificity in people with established disease (Taylor et al. 2014).

Given the limitations of currently used classification criteria, new criteria were developed using a data-driven and decision-analytic approach. These criteria have been endorsed by the American College of Rheumatology (ACR) and the European League Against Rheumatism (EULAR) and were published in 2015 (Neogi et al. 2015). The 2015 criteria are shown in Table 12.1.

Table 12.1 The 2015 ACR-EULAR gout classification criteria

Entry Criterion (Only apply criteria below to those meeting this entry criterion)		**At least one episode of swelling, pain, or tenderness in a peripheral joint or bursa**	Y/N
Sufficient Criterion (If met, can classify as gout without applying criteria below)		**Presence of MSU crystals in a symptomatic joint or bursa (i.e. in synovial fluid) or tophus**	Y/N
Criteria (to be used if Sufficient Criterion not met): *Score ≥8 required for classification as gout*		**Categories**	**Score**
CLINICAL	**Pattern of joint/bursa involvement during symptomatic* episode(s) ever**	Joint(s) or bursa(e) other than ankle, midfoot or 1st MTP (or their involvement only as part of a polyarticular presentation)	0
		Ankle OR midfoot (as part of monoarticular or oligoarticular episode)	1
		MTP1 (as part of monoarticular or oligoarticular episode)	2
	Characteristics of symptomatic episode(s) ever: Erythema overlying affected joint (patient-reported or physician-observed) can't bear touch or pressure to affected joint great difficulty with walking or inability to use affected joint	No characteristics	0
		One characteristic	1
		Two characteristics	2
		Three characteristics	3
	Time course of episode(s) ever: Presence (ever) of ≥2, irrespective of anti-inflammatory treatment: Time to maximal pain <24 hours Resolution of symptoms in ≤14 days Complete resolution (to baseline level) between symptomatic episodes	No typical episodes	0
		One typical episode	1
		Recurrent typical episodes	2
	Clinical evidence of tophus: Draining or chalk-like subcutaneous nodule under transparent skin, often with overlying vascularity, located in typical locations: joints, ears, olecranon bursae, finger pads, tendons (e.g. Achilles).	Absent	0
		Present	4

LAB	**Serum urate:** Measured by uricase method. Ideally should be scored at a time when the patient was not taking urate-lowering treatment and patient was beyond 4 weeks of the start of an episode (i.e. during intercritical period); ***if*** practicable, retest under those conditions. The highest value irrespective of timing should be scored.	<4 mg/dL [<0.24 mmol/L]	–4
		4–<6 mg/dL [0.24–<0.36 mmol/L]	0
		6–<8 mg/dL [0.36–<0.48 mmol/L]	2
		8–<10 mg/dL [0.48–<0.60 mmol/L]	3
		≥10 mg/dL [≥0.60 mmol/L]	4
	Synovial fluid analysis of a symptomatic (ever) joint or bursa: Should be assessed by a trained observer.	Not done	0
		MSU negative	–2
IMAGING‡	**Imaging evidence of urate deposition in symptomatic (ever) joint or bursa:** Ultrasound evidence of double contour sign¶ ***or*** DECT demonstrating urate deposition§.	Absent OR Not done	0
		Present (either modality)	4
	Imaging evidence of gout-related joint damage: Conventional radiography of the hands and/or feet demonstrate at least one erosion.‡	Absent OR Not done	0
		Present	4
TOTAL SCORE			
SCORE ≥ 8 = CLASSIFY AS GOUT			

*Symptomatic episodes are periods of symptoms that include any of swelling, pain, or tenderness in a peripheral joint or bursa.

¶Hyperechoic irregular enhancement over the surface of the hyaline cartilage that is independent of the insonation angle of the ultrasound beam (note: false positive DCS (artefact) may appear at the cartilage surface that should disappear with a change in the insonation angle of the probe) (Filippucci et al. 2012; Naredo et al. 2014).

§Presence of colour-coded urate at articular or periarticular sites. Images should be acquired using a dual energy computed tomography scanner, with data acquired at 80 and 140 kV and analyzed using gout-specific software with a two material decomposition algorithm which colour-codes urate (Glazebrook et al. 2011). A positive scan is defined as the presence of colour-coded urate at articular or periarticular sites. Nailbed, submillimeter, skin, motion, beam hardening, and vascular artefacts should not be interpreted as evidence of DECT urate deposition (Mallinson et al. 2014).

‡Erosion is defined as a cortical break with sclerotic margin and overhanging edge; excluding DIP joints and gull wing appearance.

Source: Reproduced from Neogi et al. (2015) with permission.

Specific points require emphasis. In order for classification as gout to be considered, at least one episode of peripheral joint or bursal swelling, pain, or tenderness is required (entry criterion). If monosodium urate (MSU) crystals are present in a symptomatic joint or bursa (i.e. synovial fluid) or in a tophus, this is considered sufficient for gout classification; no further scoring is needed.

If microscopic examination is negative or not done, other domains are considered. These domains include clinical (pattern of joint or bursa involvement, characteristics, time course of symptomatic episodes, presence of subcutaneous tophus), laboratory (serum urate, MSU-negative synovial fluid aspirate), and imaging (double contour sign on ultrasound or urate on dual energy CT, radiographic gout-related erosion). The categories are scored to a maximum score of 23. A threshold score of ≥8 classifies an individual as having gout. It is noteworthy that two categories (synovial fluid MSU-crystal-negative and serum urate <0.24 mmol/L) elicit negative scores. Compared to MSU crystal identification by microscopy as gold standard, the sensitivity and specificity of the 2015 clinical criteria are high: 92% and 89%, respectively.

The criteria allow for classification of an individual as having gout regardless of whether they are experiencing an acute flare or have any concomitant diseases. It is important to emphasize that the purpose of gout classification criteria is to define cases of gout for the purposes of research. These criteria are not intended for gout diagnosis in clinical practice. A web-based calculator is available at http://goutclassificationcalculator.auckland.ac.nz.

12.2 OMERACT-endorsed outcome measure domains and instruments for acute and chronic gout studies

The Outcomes in Rheumatology Clinical Trials (OMERACT) group has endorsed a number of outcome measure domains and instruments for use in gout clinical trials. A key development early in this process was the recognition that domains for studies of acute gout flares may be different from long-term (chronic) gout studies. Essential or mandatory domains have been identified and should be reported in all gout clinical studies (Schumacher et al. 2009). For acute gout studies, the following domains have been endorsed as mandatory: pain, joint swelling, joint tenderness, patient global assessment, and activity limitations. For chronic gout studies, the following domains have been endorsed as mandatory: serum urate, acute gout attack (flares), tophus burden, health-related quality of life (HRQOL), activity limitations, pain, and patient global assessment. A number of other discretionary domains have also been identified (Figure 12.1). At present the essential domains should be reported separately. It is currently unclear whether composite measures of disease activity are appropriate for use in gout clinical studies (Taylor et al. 2013).

For many of the essential outcome measure domains for both the acute and chronic gout studies, instruments have also been endorsed by OMERACT (Dalbeth et al. 2011b ; Singh et al. 2011; Singh et al. 2014; Stamp et al. 2011). These instruments are shown in Table 12.2.

12.3 Flare definition

Although gout flare is an essential outcome measure domain for chronic gout studies, OMERACT has not yet endorsed an instrument to measure gout flares. Provisional definitions of flare in patients with established gout (Table 12.3) have been described using a process of Delphi methodology to identify possible elements and then a multicentre international study to evaluate potential flare criteria against the gold standard of an expert rheumatologist definition (Gaffo et al. 2012). This process has identified patient-reported items of any warm joint, any swollen joint, pain at rest score of >3, and flare as key elements of the definition.

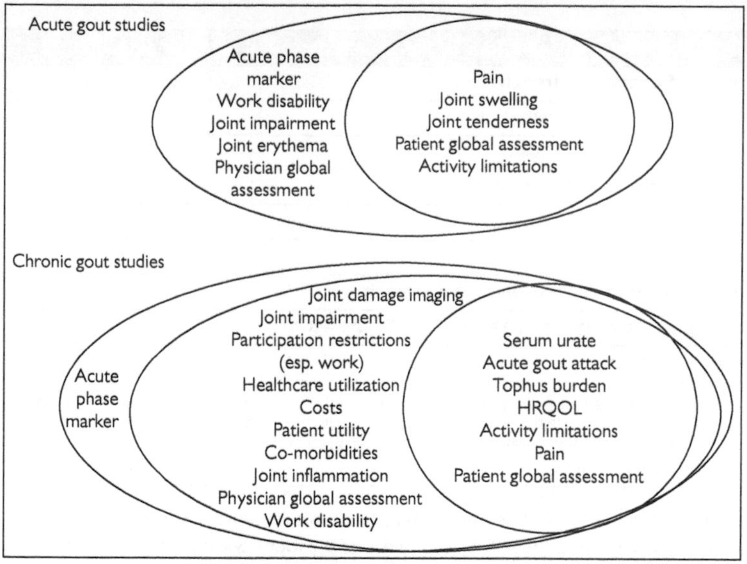

Figure 12.1 OMERACT-endorsed domains for acute and chronic gout studies.
Reprinted with permission from The Journal of Rheumatology SCHUMACHER H. R. et al, J Rheumatol 2007;34(6)

Table 12.2 Instruments endorsed by OMERACT for core domains in acute and chronic gout studies

Study type	Domain	Instrument
Acute	Pain	5-point Likert scale and/or visual analogue scale (0 to 100 mm)
	Joint swelling	4-point Likert scale for joint swelling
	Joint tenderness	4-point Likert scale for joint tenderness
	Patient global assessment	5-point Likert scale for patient global assessment of response to treatment
	Activity limitations	Nil endorsed
Chronic	Serum urate	Chemical pathology laboratory testing
	Flares	Nil endorsed
	Tophus burden	Subcutaneous index tophus maximum diameter measurement using Vernier calipers
	Health-related quality of life	Medical Outcomes Study Short-form Survey 36 (SF-36)
	Activity limitations	Health Assessment Questionnaire-Disability Index (HAQ-DI)
	Pain	Visual analogue scale for pain
	Patient global assessment	Visual analogue scale

Source: Adapted from Dalbeth et al. (2011b), Schumacher et al. (2009), Singh et al. (2011), Singh et al. (2014), and Stamp et al. (2011) with permission.

Table 12.3 Provisional definitions of flare in patients with established gout
Number-of-criteria approach
≥3 of the following four criteria:
Any patient-reported warm joint
Any patient-reported swollen joint
Patient-reported pain at rest score of >3*
Patient-reported flare
Classification-and-regression-tree approach
Patient-reported pain at rest with a score of >3*, followed by
Patient-reported flare
*Pain at rest was measured using the question, 'Considering PAIN from your gout over the last 1 week when you are RESTING (for example in bed or sitting quietly), please circle the number indicating the level of pain when it was at its WORST', using a 0 (no pain)–10 (worst imaginable pain) numerical rating scale. Source: Adapted with permission from Gaffo et al. (2012).

Two flare definitions have been proposed based on this analysis. First, using a number-of-criteria approach, the presence of three or more of the four key elements had high discrimination (sensitivity 91%, specificity 82%). Second, a classification-and-regression-tree approach identified patient-reported pain at rest with a score of >3, followed by patient self-reported flare, as the rule associated with the gold standard (sensitivity 83%, specificity 90%). These provisional flare definitions require prospective validation in independent data sets, but provide an important framework when designing and evaluating clinical trials in gout.

12.4 Gout-specific, patient-reported outcome measures

The patient-reported outcome measures currently endorsed by OMERACT for use in clinical trials are instruments used in clinical studies for a variety of rheumatic diseases (and in some cases, other non-rheumatic diseases). The characteristics of gout are quite different from other rheumatic disease, due to the fluctuating course of disease, severity of flares, and the variation of clinical presentations, ranging from occasional flares to severe chronic tophaceous gouty arthritis.

The Gout Assessment Questionnaire version 2 (GAQ2.0) is a patient-reported outcome instrument for measuring the impact of gout (Hirsch et al. 2008). It contains the gout impact section as well as sections for clinical and background data. The gout impact section is scored in five subscales: gout concern overall (four items), gout medication side effects (two items), unmet gout treatment need (three items), well-being during attack (eleven items), and gout concern during attack (four items). Each item is scored on a 5-point Likert scale. This questionnaire was developed following focus groups of people with gout and has good internal consistency and test-retest reproducibility. The GAQ2.0 correlates only modestly with generic health-related quality of life measures such as the SF-36v2. The instrument's sensitivity to change has not been conclusively demonstrated in clinical trials to date. Copies of the questionnaire are available from Takeda Pharmaceuticals.

The GAQ2.0 does not include specific questions about tophi. A patient-reported outcome instrument has also been developed for patients with tophi. The Tophus Impact Questionnaire (TIQ-20) is a publicly available 20-item questionnaire that captures core aspects of the experience of tophaceous gout (Aati et al. 2014). Developed using qualitative interviews and

Table 12.4 The Tophus Impact Questionnaire (TIQ-20)

Gouty tophi are nodules (lumps) of uric acid crystals underneath the skin. This questionnaire asks about how tophi may affect you.		
Do you have tophi?		**YES/NO**
If YES, please circle whether you agree or disagree with each statement.		
1	My tophi are painful	Agree/Disagree
2	I feel pain when my tophi are knocked	Agree/Disagree
3	I have difficulty walking because of my tophi	Agree/Disagree
4	Bending down to the ground is difficult because of my tophi	Agree/Disagree
5	Writing is difficult because of my tophi	Agree/Disagree
6	I have difficulty feeding myself because of my tophi	Agree/Disagree
7	I have to make changes to my footwear because of my tophi	Agree/Disagree
8	I have to buy special shoes because of my tophi	Agree/Disagree
9	My tophi cause financial difficulty	Agree/Disagree
10	My tophi cause difficulty participating in family life	Agree/Disagree
11	I cannot play sport because of my tophi	Agree/Disagree
12	My tophi do not have any effect on my life	Agree/Disagree
13	I feel embarrassed because of my tophi	Agree/Disagree
14	My tophi cause others to feel uncomfortable	Agree/Disagree
15	My tophi are unpleasant to look at	Agree/Disagree
16	My life would be better if I could get rid of my tophi	Agree/Disagree
17	My tophi do not bother me	Agree/Disagree
18	My tophi have become infected	Agree/Disagree
19	I have visited my doctor for treatment of my tophi	Agree/Disagree
20	I have had surgery for my tophi	Agree/Disagree

Source: Reproduced with permission from (Aati et al. 2014). A calculator for scoring is available at www.fmhs.auckland.ac.nz/TIQ-20.

Rasch analysis methodology, this instrument includes items related to pain, activity limitation, footwear modification, participation, psychological impact, and healthcare use due to tophi. The questionnaire has high face and construct validity, and acceptable test-retest reliability. Sensitivity to change has not yet been tested. The questionnaire is shown in Table 12.4. It is recommended that the Rasch-modelled TIQ-20 is reported: a scoring calculator is available at www.fmhs.auckland.ac.nz/TIQ-20.

12.5 **Imaging tools for gout research**

The properties and clinical applications of imaging methods are discussed in detail in Chapter 7. This section focuses on imaging tools used in gout research. Imaging tools may be useful for tophus measurement, an OMERACT-mandatory domain for chronic gout studies, and joint damage and inflammation, which are discretionary domains. Tophus measurement and joint damage scoring systems have been developed for gout imaging research.

For plain radiography, a modified Sharp–van der Heijde damage score, which also includes the hand distal interphalangeal joints, has been validated for gout studies (Figure 12.2) (Dalbeth et al. 2007a). This scoring system includes scoring of bone erosion and joint space narrowing, and has high face, construct, and criterion validity. The system has excellent inter-reader reproducibility, and sensitivity to change has been demonstrated in a small study of patients treated with pegloticase (Dalbeth et al. 2014).

Ultrasonography (US) can capture many aspects of disease in gout, including urate deposition, joint damage, and inflammation. Urate deposition can be assessed by the presence of the double contour sign or tophus size. US tophus measurement is highly correlated with MRI values, and is sensitive to change in response to urate-lowering therapy (Perez-Ruiz et al. 2007). Scoring systems are currently under development for US (Bruyn et al. 2015).

MRI allows volume assessment of tophi, with moderate reproducibility. Contrast is not required for MRI tophus measurement. The Rheumatoid Arthritis Magnetic Resonance Imaging System (RAMRIS) bone erosion scoring system has been used for gout MRI scans, with high inter-reader reproducibility for bone erosion (McQueen et al. 2014). A Gout MRI Cartilage Score (GOMRICS) has also been developed which is highly correlated with the total SvdH score and the joint space narrowing component, and has moderate inter-reader reliability (Popovich et al. 2014). To date, there are no data showing sensitivity to change using MRI measures.

Conventional CT allows excellent definition of bone erosions and an erosion scoring system has been developed to assess bone erosion in the feet of people with gout (Figure 12.3) (Dalbeth et al. 2011a). This system involves semi-quantitative analysis of bone erosion at seven bones in each foot. This system has high face validity and excellent inter-reader reproducibility. Sensitivity to change has not yet been reported. Tophus volume can also be measured using conventional CT. This method involves manual outlining of serial axial slices, which is labour intensive (Dalbeth et al. 2007b). CT tophus volume correlates highly with physical measurement of tophi using Vernier calipers, and for feasibility reasons, physical measurement is preferred (Dalbeth et al. 2011b).

Dual energy CT (DECT) allows analysis of bone erosion as described for conventional CT, and allows assessment of the presence and volume of urate deposits (see Chapter 7) (Choi et al. 2009). DECT allows automated volume assessments of urate deposits within regions of interest, with excellent inter-reader reliability (Choi et al. 2009; Dalbeth et al. 2012).

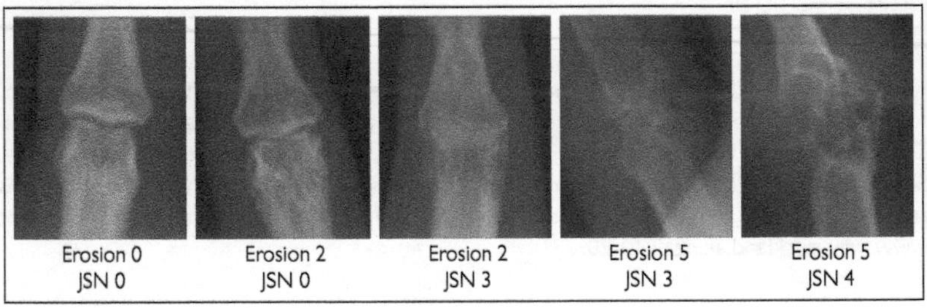

Figure 12.2 Examples of erosion and joint space narrowing (JSN) scores in proximal interphalangeal joints affected by gout.

Reused from Dalbeth, N. et al. (2007a), Validation of a radiographic damage index in chronic gout, Arthritis Rheum, 57 (6), 1067-73 with permission from John Wiley and Sons.

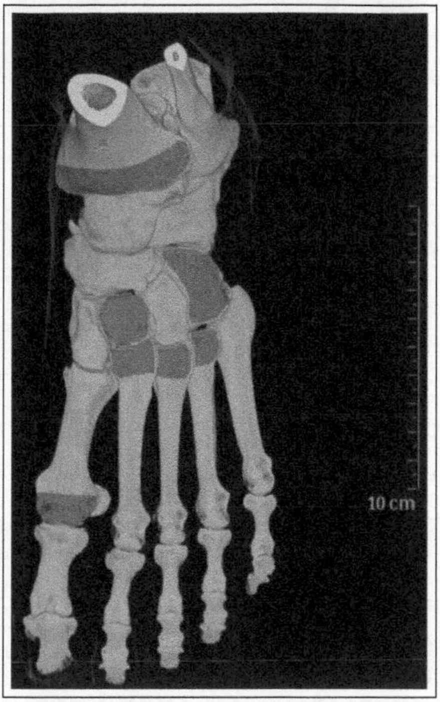

Figure 12.3 Sites for CT bone erosion scoring system.

Nicola Dalbeth et al, Development of a computed tomography method of scoring bone erosion in patients with gout: validation and clinical implications, Rheumatology, 2011, Vol 50, No. 2, by permission of Oxford University Press.

References

Aati O, et al. (2014). Development of a patient-reported outcome measure of tophus burden: the Tophus Impact Questionnaire (TIQ-20). *Annals of the Rheumatic Diseases* (early online).

Bruyn GA, et al. (2015). The OMERACT Ultrasound Working Group 10 years on: update at OMERACT 12. *Journal of Rheumatology* (early online).

Choi HK, et al. (2009). Dual energy computed tomography in tophaceous gout. *Annals of the Rheumatic Diseases*, 68(10), 1609–12.

Dalbeth N, et al. (2007a). Validation of a radiographic damage index in chronic gout. *Arthritis & Rheumatism*, 57(6), 1067–73.

Dalbeth N, et al. (2007b). Computed tomography measurement of tophus volume: comparison with physical measurement. *Arthritis & Rheumatism*, 57(3), 461–5.

Dalbeth N, et al. (2012). Assessment of tophus size: a comparison between physical measurement methods and dual-energy computed tomography scanning. *Journal of Clinical Rheumatology*, 18(1), 23–7.

Dalbeth N, et al. (2011a). Development of a computed tomography method of scoring bone erosion in patients with gout: validation and clinical implications. *Rheumatology (Oxford)*, 50(2), 410–6.

Dalbeth N, et al. (2011b). Tophus measurement as an outcome measure for clinical trials of chronic gout: progress and research priorities. *Journal of Rheumatology*, 38(7), 1458–61.

Dalbeth N, et al. (2014). Exploratory study of radiographic change in patients with tophaceous gout treated with intensive urate-lowering therapy. *Arthritis Care & Research (Hoboken)*, 66(1), 82–5.

Filippucci E, Di Geso L, Grassi W (2012). Tips and tricks to recognize microcrystalline arthritis. *Rheumatology (Oxford)*, 51(Suppl 7), vii18–21.

Gaffo AL, et al. (2012). Developing a provisional definition of flare in patients with established gout. *Arthritis & Rheumatism*, 64(5), 1508–17.

Glazebrook K N, et al. (2011). Identification of intraarticular and periarticular uric acid crystals with dual-energy CT: initial evaluation. *Radiology*, 261(2), 516–24.

Hirsch JD, et al. (2008). Evaluation of an instrument assessing influence of gout on health-related quality of life. *Journal of Rheumatology*, 35(12), 2406–14.

Mallinson PI, et al. (2014). Artifacts in dual-energy CT gout protocol: a review of 50 suspected cases with an artifact identification guide. *AJR American Journal of Roentgenology*, 203(1), W103–9.

McQueen FM, et al. (2014). Bone erosions in patients with chronic gouty arthropathy are associated with tophi but not bone oedema or synovitis: new insights from a 3 T MRI study. *Rheumatology (Oxford)*, 53(1), 95–103.

Naredo E, et al. (2014). Ultrasound-detected musculoskeletal urate crystal deposition: which joints and what findings should be assessed for diagnosing gout? *Annals of the Rheumatic Diseases*, 73(8), 1522–8.

Neogi T, et al. (2015). 2015 gout classification criteria: an American College of Rheumatology/European League Against Rheumatism collaborative initiative. *Arthritis & Rheumatology*, 67(10), 2557–2568.

Perez-Ruiz F, Martin I, Canteli B (2007). Ultrasonographic measurement of tophi as an outcome measure for chronic gout. *Journal of Rheumatology*, 34(9), 1888–93.

Popovich I, et al. (2014). Exploring cartilage damage in gout using 3-T MRI: distribution and associations with joint inflammation and tophus deposition. *Skeletal Radiology*, 43(7), 917–24.

Schumacher HR, et al. (2007). Outcome evaluations in gout. *Journal of Rheumatology*, 34(6), 1381–5.

Schumacher HR, et al. (2009). Outcome domains for studies of acute and chronic gout. *Journal of Rheumatology*, 36(10), 2342–5.

Singh JA, et al. (2011). Patient-reported outcomes in chronic gout: a report from OMERACT 10. *Journal of Rheumatology*, 38(7), 1452–7.

Singh JA, et al. (2014). OMERACT endorsement of measures of outcome for studies of acute gout. *Journal of Rheumatology*, 41(3), 569–73.

Stamp LK, et al. (2011). Serum urate in chronic gout--will it be the first validated soluble biomarker in rheumatology? *Journal of Rheumatology*, 38(7), 1462–6.

Taylor WJ, et al. (2013). Do patient preferences for core outcome domains for chronic gout studies support the validity of composite response criteria? *Arthritis Care & Research (Hoboken)*, 65(8), 1259–64.

Taylor WJ, et al. (2014). Performance of classification criteria for gout in early and established disease. *Annals of the Rheumatic Diseases*. doi:10.1136/annrheumdis-2014-206364

Wallace SL, et al. (1977). Preliminary criteria for the classification of the acute arthritis of primary gout. *Arthritis & Rheumatism*, 20(3), 895–900.

Chapter 13

The future of gout management

Key points

- At present, despite the increasing prevalence of the disease, gout is poorly treated.
- Alternative models of care within primary care offer new opportunities for effective gout management.
- In addition to more effective use of approved agents, future gout management will be improved with increasing availability of new urate-lowering drugs.
- The role of urate-lowering therapy for asymptomatic hyperuricaemia, particularly in the context of co-morbid conditions such as chronic kidney disease, hypertension, and coronary artery disease is currently unknown; large clinical trials are needed to address this key question.
- Wider and earlier adoption of urate-lowering therapy in those with established gout is likely to reduce the long-term impact of this common condition.

Gout management is currently limited by outdated attitudes to the disease and inadequate management. Although treatment targets are embedded in management guidelines, most people with gout are not currently receiving optimal treatment and do not achieve these targets. Numerous studies from many different countries have demonstrated low rates of urate-lowering therapy prescription, infrequent serum urate monitoring, suboptimal dosing of urate-lowering therapy, and poor attainment of serum urate targets in those who do have urate testing. Consequently, gout remains a painful and disabling condition that causes work absences, activity limitation, and joint damage.

Despite the current gloomy situation, the field of gout biology and therapeutics has rapidly advanced in the last decade, with important implications for clinical management. First, it is clear that gout prevalence is increasing, due to increasing survival from co-morbid conditions, such as cardiovascular disease and chronic kidney disease. The widespread availability within modern culture of sugar-sweetened beverages and alcohol, caloric excess, and purine-rich foods, together with high rates of central obesity and metabolic syndrome, further increase the population prevalence of hyperuricaemia and subsequent gout.

Gout is a condition mainly treated in primary care; new models of care to effectively manage the increasing prevalence of disease have emerged. Very high rates (>80%) of serum urate target attainment have been described in clinical situations, such as nurse-led clinics and pharmacist-based management plans, primarily using allopurinol dose-escalation strategies (Goldfien et al. 2014; Rees et al. 2013). These models represent an important advance in sustainable healthcare delivery to increasing numbers of people with gout.

Although microscopic identification of monosodium urate (MSU) crystals is the gold standard, gout remains primarily a clinical diagnosis. Non-invasive imaging methods, such as ultrasonography and dual energy CT, are important advances, and will be utilized increasingly in the future for non-invasive diagnosis. New methods of in vivo crystal identification, including

Table 13.1 Pipeline agents for urate-lowering therapy

Agent	Alternate name	Mode of action	Development stage	Potential use
Lesinurad	RDEA594	Uricosuric	Phase 3	Urate-lowering therapy
Extended release febuxostat		Xanthine oxidase inhibitor	Phase 3	Urate-lowering therapy
Ulodesine	BCX4208	Purine nucleoside phosphorylase inhibitor	Phase 2	Urate-lowering therapy
RDEA3170		Uricosuric	Phase 2	Urate-lowering therapy
KUX-1151		Xanthine oxidase inhibitor and uricosuric	Phase 2	Urate-lowering therapy
Levotofisopam		Uricosuric	Phase 2	Urate-lowering therapy
Tranilast		Uricosuric and anti-inflammatory	Phase 2	Urate-lowering therapy / gout flare prophylaxis
Arhalofenate	MBX-102	Uricosuric and IL-1β inhibition	Phase 2	Urate-lowering therapy / gout flare prophylaxis
AC-201		Uricosuric and IL-1β inhibition	Phase 2	Urate-lowering therapy / gout flare prophylaxis
RLBN1001 and analogues		Xanthine oxidase inhibitor and uricosuric	Proof of concept	Urate-lowering therapy

Source: http://www.ClinicalTrials.gov (accessed March 2015).

Raman spectroscopy, offer further promise for accurate, non-invasive diagnosis without the need for ionizing radiation.

More than ten urate-lowering agents are available in pipeline development as urate-lowering therapy in people with gout. These agents are summarized in Table 13.1, based on a search of http://www.ClinicalTrials.gov. Several of these agents are proposed to have anti-inflammatory effects, which might allow a dual action of both urate-lowering therapy and prophylaxis against gout flares. Such therapies would have major clinical benefit, as flares during initiation of urate-lowering drugs are a frequent cause for patients with gout stopping these agents, and avoiding future use.

In addition to new therapies, better use of approved urate-lowering drugs is required for future gout management. Currently there is a reluctance to use effective doses of drugs such as allopurinol or febuxostat, and older uricosuric agents, such as probenecid, are very infrequently used (Singh et al. 2015). When prescribed according to serum urate targets up to maximum approved doses, these agents are highly effective at achieving serum urate levels required to promote urate crystal dissolution, reduce flares, and regress tophi. New trials that examine the best dosing strategies for approved drugs in real-life clinical practice will lead to improved and cost-effective gout management within primary care.

At present, urate-lowering therapy is recommended for those with established gout; namely, in those who are experiencing frequent flares or who have large burden of urate crystal deposition, with clinically apparent tophi and joint damage. The 2015 European League Against Rheumatism (EULAR) gout management guidelines suggest that urate-lowering therapy should be considered in patients with gout after the first flare of disease. The recognition that MSU crystals are present on advanced imaging in some hyperuricaemic individuals even before onset of symptomatic disease raises the possibility that some people with asymptomatic hyperuricaemia may benefit from urate-lowering therapy. This may be particularly relevant in patients with conditions associated with hyperuricaemia, such as hypertension, chronic kidney disease, and coronary artery disease. The benefits and risks of urate-lowering therapy in asymptomatic hyperuricaemia, with or without subclinical urate crystal deposits, are currently unknown, and future studies will clarify the patient acceptability and therapeutic role of such an approach.

Despite the uncertainty regarding urate-lowering therapy for asymptomatic hyperuricaemia, the use of urate-lowering therapy for those with symptomatic gout is well established. Current perceptions of the gout as a self-inflicted disease caused by dietary excess and gluttony leads to social stigma in the wider community and a focus on dietary management as the key component of gout treatment by healthcare professionals (Lindsay et al. 2011). Scientific advances demonstrating the genetic basis of the disease and the importance of renal urate transporters in the pathogenesis of disease should translate into destigmatization and a shift in the perception of gout to a disease of disordered urate transport. Such a change in attitudes in both healthcare professionals and within the general community—together with widening treatment options and increasing success in gout management—should ultimately lead to improved treatment of gout. Increased use of effective urate-lowering therapy, prior to onset of tophi and joint damage, will reduce the impact of inadequately treated gout in the community.

References

Goldfien RD, et al. (2014). Effectiveness of a pharmacist-based gout care management programme in a large integrated health plan: results from a pilot study *BMJ Open*, 4(1), e003627.

Lindsay K, et al. (2011). The experience and impact of living with gout: a study of men with chronic gout using a qualitative grounded theory approach *Journal of Clinical Rheumatology*, 17(1), 1–6.

Rees F, Jenkins W, Doherty M (2013). Patients with gout adhere to curative treatment if informed appropriately: proof-of-concept observational study *Annals of the Rheumatic Diseases*, 72(6), 826–30.

Singh JA, Akhras KS, Shiozawa A (2015). Comparative effectiveness of urate lowering with febuxostat versus allopurinol in gout: analyses from large US managed care cohort *Arthritis Research & Therapy*, 17(1), 120.

Index